TREATING SEXUAL DESIRE DISORDERS

Treating Sexual Desire Disorders

A Clinical Casebook

Edited by

SANDRA R. LEIBLUM

THE GUILFORD PRESS
New York   London

© 2010 The Guilford Press
A Division of Guilford Publications, Inc.
72 Spring Street, New York, NY 10012
www.guilford.com

Printed in the United States of America

This book is printed on acid-free paper.

Last digit is print number: 9 8 7 6 5 4 3 2 1

The authors have checked with sources believed to be reliable in their efforts to provide
information that is complete and generally in accord with the standards of practice
that are accepted at the time of publication. However, in view of the possibility of
human error or changes in medical sciences, neither the authors, nor the editor and
publisher, nor any other party who has been involved in the preparation or publication
of this work warrants that the information contained herein is in every respect accurate
or complete, and they are not responsible for any errors or omissions or the results
obtained from the use of such information. Readers are encouraged to confirm the
information contained in this book with other sources.

Library of Congress Cataloging-in-Publication Data

Leiblum, Sandra Risa.
  Treating sexual desire disorders: a clinical casebook / Sandra R. Leiblum.
    p. cm.
  Includes bibliographical references and index.
  ISBN 978-1-60623-636-9 (hard cover: alk. paper)
  1. Sex therapy. 2. Sexual disorders—treatment. I. Title.
  RC557.L35 2010
  616.85′8306—dc22

                                                    2010001285

IN MEMORIAM
Sandra R. Leiblum (1943–2010)

Sandy Leiblum, born in Brooklyn, New York, and never without that distinctive accent, was a true sexology star. She contributed some of the most important books to the field over a period of decades, specializing in clinical compilations that showed the diversity of treatment approaches to a wide variety of sexual problems. Much of her experience came from decades of teaching and mentoring young psychology and medical colleagues in New Jersey. Sandy was an active participant in and was repeatedly elected president of the leading professional organizations in the field, receiving all their important honors. She pioneered the recognition of persistent genital arousal as a problem. She wrote swiftly, and with clarity. She was an excellent friend and collaborator to many of us and a superb mother to Jonathan (Jake). Her death was unexpected and far too soon. Sandy was involved in many important professional developments and was at the height of professional recognition. She is mourned by her husband, Frank, and by her numerous friends in the United States and around the world. A bright star, a snappy dresser, a warm and loving friend, is gone.

About the Editor

Sandra R. Leiblum, PhD, was, until her death in January 2010, Professor of Psychiatry and Obstetrics/Gynecology, Director of the Center for Sexual and Relationship Health, and Director of the Psychology Internship Program at the Robert Wood Johnson Medical School, University of Medicine and Dentistry of New Jersey, in Piscataway, New Jersey. An internationally recognized authority in sex therapy, Dr. Leiblum received numerous awards for her professional contributions, including the Masters and Johnson Award from the Society for Sex Therapy and Research and the Professional Standard of Excellence Award from the American Association of Sexuality Educators, Counselors and Therapists. She was the author or editor of over 125 journal articles, chapters, and books on various aspects of male and female sexuality and was widely recognized for her teaching and clinical activities. Her book *Principles and Practice of Sex Therapy, Fourth Edition* (Guilford, 2006) received the 2010 SSTAR Health Professional Book Award from the Society for Sex Therapy and Research.

Contributors

Rosemary Basson, MD, Sexual Medicine Clinic, Vancouver General Hospital, Vancouver, British Columbia, Canada

Alisa Breetz, MA, Department of Psychology, American University, Washington, DC

Lori A. Brotto, PhD, Department of Obstetrics and Gynaecology, University of British Columbia, Vancouver, British Columbia, Canada

Irwin Goldstein, MD, San Diego Sexual Medicine, Alvarado Hospital, San Diego, California

Sue W. Goldstein, BA, San Diego Sexual Medicine, Alvarado Hospital, San Diego, California

Kathryn Hall, PhD, private practice, Princeton, New Jersey

Marny Hall, PhD, private practice, Oakland, California

Peggy J. Kleinplatz, PhD, Faculty of Medicine and School of Psychology, University of Ottawa, Ottawa, Ontario, Canada

Joanna B. Korda, MD, San Diego Sexual Medicine, Alvarado Hospital, San Diego, California

Michael Krychman, MD, private practice, Newport Beach, California

Sandra R. Leiblum, PhD (deceased), Department of Psychiatry and Obstetrics/Gynecology, Center for Sexual and Relationship Health, and Psychology Internship Program, Robert Wood Johnson Medical School, University of Medicine and Dentistry of New Jersey, Piscataway, New Jersey

Barry McCarthy, PhD, Washington Psychological Center, Washington, DC

Esther Perel, MA, LMFT, private practice, New York, New York

Bonnie R. Saks, MD, Department of Psychiatry, University of South Florida, Tampa, Florida

David Schnarch, PhD, Marriage and Family Health Center of Evergreen Colorado, Evergreen, Colorado

Douglas K. Snyder, PhD, Department of Psychology, Texas A&M University, College Station, Texas

Susan Kellogg Spadt, PhD, Pelvic and Sexual Health Institute, Philadelphia, Pennsylvania

Leonore Tiefer, PhD, Department of Psychiatry, New York University School of Medicine, New York, New York

David C. Treadway, PhD, private practice, Weston, Massachusetts

Jane S. T. Woo, MA, Department of Psychology, University of British Columbia, Vancouver, British Columbia, Canada

Preface

There is no shortage of advice in bookstores and on media talk shows for bolstering sagging sex drives: Pop some steamy porn on the TV or computer, blindfold or bind a mate to the headboard, arrange a weekend or night in a no-tell motel, titillate a vagina or massage a phallus with sensual oils, and so forth. While these nostrums might work once or twice or maybe even for a whole week, once the novelty wears off, so does the interest in sex. The sad truth is, once couples fall out of the habit of regular sexual connection, it is difficult to revive—and can explain the appeal of new relationships or a change of partners. For most couples in long-term partnerships, particularly those in which one partner has low, modest, or absent sexual desire and the other does not, the challenge of reawakening or creating desire is considerable. While it is certainly true that the experience of sexual arousal may whet desire, the knowledge that this is so does not always lead folks to the conjugal bed. As clinicians, we are constantly faced with the challenge of helping frustrated, thwarted, and disappointed partners with complaints about their own or their partner's sexual apathy. This is not always easy or successful.

These are the reasons for undertaking this book: to acknowledge the difficulty couples experience and to benefit from the wisdom of expert clinicians who encounter these issues daily. How do clinicians deal with the most prevalent sexual complaint of all—what has been christened with the sanitized name *hypoactive sexual desire disorder*, or HSDD? There are few long-term outcome studies of the successful treatment of HSDD, unlike the impressive research literature that has accumulated on the treatment of orgasmic disorders or erectile problems. It is far more common for clinicians to bemoan their failures than to boast of their successes with these cases. Yet now, more than ever, we are seeing a parade of both men and women complaining of sexual apathy despite good health, good will, and even good relationships.

In the chapters that follow, the reader will discover sage advice and sound interventions for working with individuals and couples who are struggling with desire issues. While not promising total success, many contributors report significant improvement with treatment. The complexity and diversity of these cases will illustrate how varied the etiological and maintaining factors that characterize these cases are and why, realistically, there can be no single treatment approach.

As a clinician myself, I am very grateful to the impressive and worthy group of authors who were willing to participate in this project. All are busy and successful professionals with a host of other commitments, yet each of them was willing to take the time to think about and articulate his or her approach to treating desire problems. And I hope you too, as a reader, will find much to enlighten and assist you in working with these most challenging problems.

SANDRA R. LEIBLUM

Note: Sandra R. Leiblum suffered a devastating accident after the manuscript had been sent to the publisher. She died in January 2010. Leonore Tiefer, one of the contributors and a long-time friend, agreed to shepherd the manuscript through the final editorial stages.

Contents

Chapter 1

Introduction and Overview

Clinical Perspectives on and Treatment for Sexual Desire Disorders

Sandra R. Leiblum

Sexual desire is the most elusive of passions. While easily ignited in a new relationship or a forbidden encounter, it can also be readily extinguished. Anxiety, hostility, bad memories, or frightening flashbacks can thwart it—even something as simple as the sound of a door opening or a child crying. And yet, when aroused by an image or scent or fantasy or person, it can feel powerfully intense, driven, lively, and life-affirming. Interest in and concerns about absent or diminished desire have never, perhaps, been greater.

Historically, sexual desire has rarely been viewed from a neutral or disinterested stance. Attempts have always been made either to stimulate libido—whether through perfumes, potions, prostitutes, or pictures—or to stifle it. Whereas in previous decades, sexual complaints may have centered on "performance"—erectile or orgasmic problems—in the recent past, concerns about sexual *desire* have become paramount. There are several reasons for this.

An active and satisfying sexual life is widely regarded not only as desirable but as a sign of emotional and physical health. When desire ebbs, intimate connections seem to diminish as well. Many sexually apathetic individuals worry that their partners will look elsewhere for sexual stimulation or gratification. There is no shortage of technological options for satisfying sexual curiosity and piquing sexual arousal. The availability of pro-erection drugs, arousal creams and gels, vibrators and massage oils provides frequent reminders that sex can and should be part of life. The sexually disinterested person is made to feel deficient, dissatisfied, or dysfunctional. This pressure to conform to current norms has led a growing group of women and men to believe that if they no longer experience sexual interest or desire, something is wrong with *them* rather than with their expectations or with their partner or with society's (and the media's) ever-constant preoccupation with sex.

WHAT IS SEXUAL DESIRE?

For most people, the concept of sexual desire conjures up visions of an energizing force that motivates one to seek out or initiate genital expression and relief. Like hunger or thirst, the so-called sexual "drive" has been regarded traditionally as an instinctive, spontaneous, and insistent source of sexual motivation. It was believed to dwell within the individual and to be biologically based. Linked to this idea is the antiquated belief that if the so-called sexual drive is not permitted free expression, it will seek an outlet through other means. The "drive reduction" model of sexual desire reached its acme with Freud's (1962) libido theory. This view asserted that the primary goal of sexual expression is to relieve libidinal tension and to restore emotional equilibrium. It suggests that sexual desire is endogenous and inevitable: everyone has it, albeit in varying amounts and to various degrees. From a traditional analytic perspective, a lack of desire results from the active repression or inhibition of the spontaneous urge for sexual contact as a result of internal conflict or ambivalence.

Current thinking challenges this view in many instances, even questioning the importance of a biological basis for libido. While the androgens, particularly testosterone, are widely credited in both the professional and popular press as the hormone responsible for libido, many sexual theorists now suggest that relational, cognitive, motivational, and evaluative factors play a more significant role. In young hypogonadal men, testosterone is usually recommended for enhancing quality of life. But there has been greater controversy about the use of androgens for triggering libido in men with late-onset hypogo-nadism, principally because other conditions may be responsible for diminished sexual desire, for example diabetes mellitus, hyperpro-lactinemia, metabolic syndrome, or a host of medications (Wang et al., 2009).

In women, recent research has found that the correlation between testosterone (however measured) and various parameters of sexual behavior is far from clear (Davis, Davison, Donath, & Bell, 2005). While there are several good studies supporting the use of androgen supplementation for increasing desire both in natural and in surgically post-menopausal women (Shifren et al., 2000; Buster et al., 2004; Simon et al., 2005), there is also sound research ques-tioning the significance of serum levels of androgen in motivating sexual behavior (Davis et al., 2005). Given that androgen levels are extremely low in women and difficult to measure precisely, the role of androgens in female sexual drive is hotly debated. At this time, there are no testosterone products approved by the Food and Drug Administration (FDA) that are available for women in the United States, although such products are available for men. While it is beyond the scope of this chapter to review the ongoing controversy surrounding the role of testosterone in stimulating libido, many of the authors in the chapters that follow address this issue in more detail. In particular, Korda, Goldstein, and Goldstein (Chapter 12) discuss the successful use of androgenic therapy in their treatment of a young woman presenting with a chronic lack of both desire and arousal. Basson (Chapter 8) presents a more cautionary view of the conclusions that may be drawn from the current research on andro-gens and sexuality.

Certainly, a serious flaw in the "drive" theory of desire is the erroneous belief that the internal or spontaneous experience of desire is not only ubiquitous but a necessary prerequisite to the experience of sexual arousal. In fact, several sex researchers persuasively argue the opposite, namely, that desire is more often secondary to arousal. It is the awareness of arousal, whether genital or subjective, that is basic in both triggering and maintaining sexual desire. This position has been eloquently articulated and described by Basson (2001) in her reformulation of the sexual response cycle, although many theorists prior to Basson emphasized the importance of arousability and exter-nal motivation as triggers for sexual desire (Beach, 1956; Whalen, 1966).

Finally, there is a growing awareness of *asexuality*, or the absence of sexual desire or interest, as a normative and legitimate life style and sexual orientation for some women and some men (Bogaert, 2004, 2006). A 1977 paper by Johnson entitled "Asexual and Autoerotic Women: Two Invisible Groups," defined asexuals as those men and women "who, regardless of physical or emotional condition, actual sexual history, and marital status or ideological orientation, *prefer* not to engage in sexual activity." Johnson (1977) contrasted auto-erotic women with asexual women: the latter are said to have no sexual desires at all, whereas the "autoerotic woman … recognizes such desires but prefers to satisfy them alone." Johnson's evidence is quite tenuous, consisting mostly of letters to the editors of women's magazines. However, her theorizing concerning asexuality as a distinct sexual orientation received support from analysis of a pro-vocative question included as part of a large-scale survey of more than 18,000 British men and women that was conducted in 2004. A professor at Brock University in Canada, Anthony Bogaert, exam-ined their answers to a question regarding sexual attraction to others, one of whose choices was "I have never felt attracted to anyone at all." He found that about 1% of the respondents reported having no sexual attraction to anyone. While it is unclear whether asexuality represents a distinct sexual orientation, like homosexuality or het-erosexuality, or whether it simply represents a variant of hypoactive sexual desire disorder, it is interesting that an online community has developed around the legitimacy of asexuality as a normal lifestyle of healthy but sexually disinterested individuals. There is even an online community and support organization, the *Asexual Visibility and Education Network (AVEN)*, founded in 2001 with two primary goals: to create public acceptance and discussion of asexuality and to facilitate the growth of an asexual community.

The authors of the chapters that follow provide many defini-tions and theories of sexual desire, its wellsprings, and its mutations. Despite the passage of more than 20 years, a definition of sexual desire presented in the 1988 edition of *Sexual Desire Disorders* (Leiblum & Rosen) still makes some intuitive sense—namely, a view of desire as a subjective and motivating feeling state triggered by both internal and external cues, which may or may not result in overt sexual behavior. Adequate neuroendocrine function seem to be essential for this feeling state to occur, along with exposure to sufficiently intense sexual stim-uli, cues, and motives or incentives. These arise from sources within the individual (a stimulating fantasy, a decision or wish to please a partner, an awareness of genital vasocongestion) but also from the environment—sexy words and provocative touch over a candlelit dinner; a photo of a restrained woman in 6-inch heels and little else; a man in tight briefs with a silky whip. Furthermore, sexual desire appears to be readily conditioned and "scripted" to socially sanctioned as well as to socially proscribed cues. Not surprisingly, in light of this last observation, we are now seeing an ever-increasing number of men and women who have been labeled as sex "addicts" for their obsessive and, at times, compulsive pursuit of both conventional and unconventional sex. It is interesting that concerns about excessive sexual interest (*hypersexual* desire) have now joined the litany of sexual complaints presented to sex therapists.

Finally, it must be acknowledged that the motivations or incentives to either initiate or respond to a sexual invitation or overture are quite varied. In a clever and provocative research study conducted by Meston and Buss (2007), 237 possible reasons for having sex were collected. These ranged from the spiritual ("I wanted to get closer to God") to the instrumental ("I wanted to experience physical pleasure"). A large sample of undergraduates ($N = 1,549$) were asked to evaluate the degree to which each of the 237 reasons led them to have sexual intercourse. Using factor analysis, four main factors and 13 subfactors emerged: *Physical* (stress reduction, pleasure, physical desirability, and experience seeking), *Goal attainment* (resources, social status, revenge, and utilitarian), and *Emotional* reasons (love and commitment and emotional expression). The three *Insecurity* subfactors were elevation of self-esteem, duty/pressure, and mate guarding.

Past research has repeatedly demonstrated that desire, arousal, and the presence or absence of sexual behavior do not always coincide in women. In 2003, Weijmar Schultz and Van de Wiel observed that despite reports of negative genital sensations, pain, and diminished desire from women who had undergone cervical cancer, these women were statistically no different in terms of frequency and motivation for sexual interaction from an age-matched control group. These authors wondered if women's "love ethos" made them more inclined to adapt to the wishes of their partners. Obviously, it is also possible that the threat of losing a lover as well as the threat of punishment or abuse may lead many disempowered or fearful women to acquiesce to sexual interactions, despite a lack of desire.

Obviously, knowing that a sexual experience has occurred tells us nothing about either the desire accompanying it or the diverse, and not necessarily sexual, motives for engaging in it.

SEXUAL DESIRE: TOO LITTLE, TOO MUCH, TOO DIFFERENT, OR JUST RIGHT?

In some respects, sexual desire complaints resemble the experience of the three bears entering the cottage in the woods and surveying the three beds lying within. "Too big," announces Momma Bear, when gazing at one bed; "Too small," announces Poppa Bear, testing out another; "Just right," pronounces Baby Bear, as he hops up and down on the middle bed. Though our patients are not bears (except perhaps when they become disgruntled), desire problems often fall into these categories as well—too little or too much. "Too little," or hypoactive sexual desire disorder (HSDD), is the most common complaint clinicians encounter, often delivered by a disappointed mate who wants greater sexual frequency and certainly a more enthusiastic sexual partner. "Too much" is also a complaint, typically made by a weary mate who finds himself or herself deflecting the sexual overtures of an indefatigably ardent lover. But "just right" sexual desire is rarely heard by clinicians, although it probably characterizes the majority of individuals who are basically satisfied with their sexual life. It should be pointed out that there is absolutely no frequency of sexual encounters that defines sexual "normality." Recent research (Schneidewind-Skibbe, Hayes, Koochaki, Meyer, & Dennerstein, 2008) highlights the fact that the mean frequency of sexual intercourse, to consider only one measure of sexual behavior, varies significantly cross-globally across all age groups. Higher rates are reported by European and American women and lower rates reported by Asian women. Many factors were found to be associated with these differences in intercourse frequency: age, parity, relationship duration, pregnancy, time, relationship status, fertility intentions, and use of contraception. Given the wide range of frequency reported, as well as the varying cultural and social context in which sexual behavior occurs, it would be arbitrary to establish where "normal" sexual frequency ends and pathologically low or excessive sexual activity starts. As clinicians we are most concerned not with how often or how infrequently our patients engage in sex, but rather with how concordant their sexual preferences and satisfaction are. Clinically, it is "too different" or too discrepant sexual interest that is the problem we must often address, since it is this complaint that leads to relationship discontent, disharmony, and distress.

LACK OF DESIRE: A BRIEF HISTORICAL OVERVIEW

At this juncture, someone might ask whether the attention being paid to sexual desire complaints nowadays is not misguided or excessive. Certainly, there have always been individuals who get along just fine without craving or engaging in sex. Should we even diagnose low sexual interest as a sexual dysfunction, since by so doing we may be pathologizing normal variations in sexual interest that are due to a host of sociocultural and relationship causes? This is certainly the position of Tiefer and Hall, who present their "new view" model in Chapter 7. They acknowledge that whether or not desire problems are ubiquitous, they definitely are *not* indicative of a psychiatric disorder.

Thoughts about this issue have certainly changed over the decades. One hundred years ago, excessive desire was regarded as aberrant. While permitted and even applauded in men, too much sexual desire in women was seen as worrisome. Sexually enthusiastic women ran the risk of being labeled as nymphomaniacs and treated medically.

Times have changed, of course, and today, concerns about sexual apathy are the most common complaint presented to sex therapists. Despite the widespread assumption that it is women who are shortchanged when it comes to libido, nowadays men are as likely as women to be diagnosed with HSDD as defined by the *Diagnostic and Statistical Manual of Mental Disorders* (DSM-IV-TR; American Psychiatric Association, 2000).

In fact, this is not a new diagnosis. Since the mid-1900s, low desire has been considered a psychiatric disorder and it was included as one of the five psychosexual disorders listed in DSM-III (American Psychiatric Association, 1980). In 1980, it was believed that without psychological inhibition, *all* individuals would experience "normal" desire. In DSM-IV (American Psychiatric Association, 1994), psychosexual disorders were elaborated as *disturbances in sexual desire and in the psychophysiologic changes that characterize the sexual response cycle which cause marked distress and interpersonal difficulty.* There was no attempt to specify a particular frequency of sexual behavior or activity as normative or deviant. Rather, it was left to the clinician to determine whether a condition warranted diagnosis, taking into account such factors as the age and experience of the individual, the frequency and chronicity of symptoms, the degree of subjective distress, and the impact on other areas of functioning. In addition, the clinician was advised to consider the contributions of an individual's ethnic, cultural, religious, and social background that might influence sexual desire, expectations, and attitudes about sexual performance.

In 1998, the Sexual Function Health Council of the American Foundation for Urologic Disease (AFUD) convened a consensus conference to review and update the current classification of female sexual disorders. One goal was to ensure that the diagnostic entities would be applicable in both medical and mental health settings. Another was to determine whether the current descriptions of female sexual disorders reflected clinical reality.

The conference invited a multidisciplinary group of European and North American research and clinical experts in the field of female sexuality, comprising sex therapists, sex researchers, gynecologists, urologists, and experts in sexual psychophysiology, among others. A recommendation emerged from that meeting that the DSM-IV definition of HSDD be amended to reflect the fact that many women never experience spontaneous sexual desire, but rather are *receptive to, and interested in sexual activity* once it is started.

In 2000, a second consensus meeting was held and the recommendation at that time was to rename HSDD as women's sexual interest/desire disorder and to define it as "absent or diminished feelings of sexual interest or desire, absent sexual thoughts or fantasies and a lack of responsive desire. Motivations (here defined as reasons/ incentives) for attempting to become sexually aroused are scarce or absent. The lack of interest is considered to be beyond a normative lessening with life cycle and relationship duration" (Basson et al., 2003, p. 224). Even this definition has generated controversy. It is likely that DSM-V (scheduled to be released in 2013) will offer yet another definition of low or absent sexual desire, perhaps combining it with diminished sexual arousal since it is often difficult, particularly for women, to discriminate between arousal and desire complaints.

In recent years, the voices of some who question the legitimacy of (and motives for) for diagnosing low desire have become louder and more insistent. In 2003, for example, an editorial in the *British Journal of Medicine* by Ray Moynihan unleashed a storm of controversy when he assailed and mocked the motives of those who regard, diagnose, and treat HSDD as a sexual dysfunction. Moynihan asserted that the identification of low desire as a psychiatric disorder was merely a ploy by pharmaceutical companies and naive clinicians to create a dysfunction that they might then develop a pill to treat. His article provoked much media controversy and many letters to the editor, with physicians, patients, and sex therapists supporting or refuting his allegations. Countering his remarks, for example, were letters highlighting the fact that desire complaints were identified as disorders in the DSM decades earlier and that by 1977, lack of desire was already acknowledged as a problem reported to clinicians by their patients (Kaplan, 1977; Lief, 1977; Basson & Leiblum, 2003).

Despite honest debate among clinicians and researchers as to how to define hypoactive sexual desire or whether to diagnose it as a disorder, there can be little doubt that a discrepancy of sexual interest and desire creates significant discontent and problems in the context of a relationship. While judicious and careful assessment must accompany any decision to treat desire complaints, an individual or couple experiencing genuine distress at sexual apathy and lack of arousal must be regarded as legitimately entitled to assistance.

PREVALENCE OF DESIRE DISORDERS

Although it often appears as if every sexually active person complains of sexual disinterest for some period of time, the actual prevalence of desire disorders varies widely, ranging anywhere from a low of 8% to a high of 55% (Deeks & McCabe, 2001; Richters, Grulichade Visser, Smith, & Rissel, 2001). While it is possible that some of the differences are attributable to the unique population studied (e.g., young vs. older individuals, pre- vs. postmenopausal women), much of the variation in prevalence estimates is likely due to differences in the way in which low desire is assessed (Hayes et al., 2007). In one study, for example, Hayes and his colleagues used several different instruments for determining the prevalence of a variety of female sexual dysfunctions. For HSDD, they compared estimates using the Sexual Function Questionnaire (SFQ; Quirk et al., 2002) either alone or in combination with the Female Sexual Distress Scale (FSDS; Derogatis, Rosen, Leiblum, Burnett, & Heiman, 2002), as well as two sets of simple questions concerning sexual interest that were adapted from a large-scale survey of sexual complaints (Laumann, Gagnon, Michael, & Michaels, 1994). Respondents were asked to report on sexual difficulties occurring during the previous month and on sexual difficulties lasting for at least 1 month in the previous year.

Of the 786 women who received the packet of questionnaires

assessing sexual interest, 45% completed the instruments. Of note, when assessed by the SFQ alone, 48% of the respondents reported low desire while 58% reported lack of sexual interest lasting for more than 1 month during the prior year. However, when the FSDS, which assesses distress about sexual desire or function, was included, the figures dropped dramatically. In fact, when assessed by the combined SFQ-FSDS scales, the prevalence of HSDD was only 16%! Moreover, changing the recall period from the previous month to 1 month or more during the previous year approximately doubled the prevalence estimates for all of the sexual complaints, while adding the questions about distress resulted in a nearly two-thirds reduction in prevalence estimates.

What can be learned from this study? First, how one assesses the *duration* of sexual disinterest results in very different estimates of prevalence. If women are asked about lack of desire that lasted 6 months or longer, prevalence estimates of HSDD will be lower than if asked about difficulties that lasted for 1 month or more (Mercer et al., 2003; Hayes, Bennett, Fairley, & Dennerstein, 2006). Moreover, without the experience of significant distress either on the part of the low-desire individual or the partner, it is unlikely that there will be a significant inclination to seek treatment unless the problem is causing relationship discord. Even then, it is likely that there will be ambivalent motives for altering the status quo. Typically, once a pattern of sexual avoidance or sexual apathy has become engrained, it becomes a new status quo. It is for this reason that complaints involving desire are so difficult to treat successfully—lack of desire is usually not experienced as a major problem for the low-desire individual, and many couples adapt to a "sexless" marriage even though they may bemoan the loss of sexual passion.

GENDER DIFFERENCES IN DESIRE

For centuries, it has been believed that women lack strong, resilient, and proactive sexual desire, unlike men, who are "always ready." As Maurice observes (2007, p. 183), "Men not interested in sex? To most, the idea is an oxymoron." The truth is that all women are not limpid, lustless creatures, devoid of lively libidos, and all men are not bursting with testosterone-infused sexual motivation.

In fact, contemporary clinicians report that the numbers of men who are disinterested in sex are not dissimilar from the numbers of women complaining (or accused) of having low sexual interest. Survey results of data collected during the Massachusetts Male Aging Study of 1,709 men between the ages of 40 and 70 found a "consistent and significant decline with age in feeling desire, in sexual thoughts and dreams, and in the desired level of sexual activity" (McKinlay & Feldman, 1994, p. 271). Clearly male sexual desire, like female sexual desire, declines with age. But it is not only older men who display a decline in sexual interest. Many younger men, too, are identified as lacking libido. While some of these men are secretly pursuing an active masturbatory or fantasy sexual life (as in the case described by McCarthy and Breetz in Chapter 5), it is also the case that there are men with long-standing and generalized low sexual desire. Women partnered with, or married to, such men are not only frustrated and angry, they often feel unattractive and unloved since they cannot comprehend why their partners are avoiding sexual (and, often, physical) intimacy with them. Many such women also feel thwarted in their desire to become pregnant and start a family. While women with low desire can still engage in sexual relations at the insistence of a demanding mate, or in order to forestall guilt and recrimination, men with low libido often have secondary erectile problems and cannot "deliver" sex in order to satisfy an insistent female partner.

Nevertheless, among older adults, the stereotype that women need to be coaxed, seduced, or even coerced into having sex continues to exist. Recall the Ogden Nash verse, "Candy is dandy but liquor is quicker." In fact, even today, some health professionals, frustrated by the absence of a pro-sexual magic elixir, suggest that with a little alcohol-mediated disinhibition or relaxation, women will be more sexually receptive.

Recent research has definitely challenged the notion that female sexual desire is merely a pale imitation of male desire. The work of Meredith Chivers (2005; Chivers, Rieger, Latty, & Bailey, 2004), for example, is a case in point. In a series of clever experiments, she highlighted the fact that women respond physiologically to sexual stimuli as quickly as do men, and, significantly, that they also respond genitally to a broader array of sexual images than men—images that depict both preferred and nonpreferred scenes (e.g., heterosexual and homosexual images, bonobo monkeys, exercising women, and even depictions of rape).

While Chivers believes that women's sexual desire may be more receptive than aggressive, that women may be evolutionarily programmed to have reflexive physiological arousal to a wide array of stimuli, and that their subjective sexual desire is discordant with their physiological arousal due to cultural or social constraints, others believe that intimacy is the major key to awakening female desire. Rosemary Basson (2001) is an advocate of this position. So is Lisa Diamond (2005). Diamond argues that female desire is quite malleable and is predicated more on emotional closeness than on gender. Flexibility and fluidity are viewed as the essence of female desire by Diamond, who studied the erotic attractions of nearly 100 women over 10 years. While many of these women initially self-identified as lesbian or bisexual, a decade later, two-thirds reported occasional attraction to men. Moreover, many women agreed with the statement "I'm the kind of person who becomes physically attracted to the person rather than his or her gender." While this same research has not been done with men, it is unlikely that one would find the same fluidity in terms of the *objects* of desire.

Finally, still another female sexuality researcher, Marta Meana, has suggested that being desired is the key to women's experience of desire (Bergner, 2009). She believes that female desire is essentially narcissistic—that intimacy is not as much of an aphrodisiac as being lusted after. However, she and other researchers all acknowledge that the variability of desire within genders is greater than the differences between men and women.

AGE-RELATED CHANGES IN SEXUAL DESIRE AND DISTRESS

Most studies find that *sexual desire diminishes with age* for both men and women. What is interesting is that *distress about reduced or lack of sexual desire also tends to diminish with age*. Hayes, Dennerstein, Bennett, and Fairley (2008) compared two populations of women between the ages of 20 and 70 in Europe and in the United States. For both European and American women, the complaint of low desire increased with age—the proportion of European women with lack of desire *increased* from 11% among women ages 20–29 to 53% in women ages 60–70. However, the proportion of women with low desire who were *distressed* about their low desire *decreased* with age. In the 20- to 29-year age group, 65% of European women and 67% of American women with low sexual desire were distressed by it, but these numbers decreased to 22% and 37%, respectively, in the 60- to 70-year age group. Apparently many individuals come to accept the reality that sexual desire diminishes with age and relationship duration, and there may be less distress about these changes. However, it should be noted that clinically, we continue to see men and women who regret their diminished desire and want to restore or reignite their sexual passion. In Chapter 2, Esther Perel discusses the challenges of maintaining eroticism and desire in the face of domesticity and predictability.

ETIOLOGY OF DESIRE DISORDERS

One of the challenges of treating sexual desire problems is the fact that the etiology is so varied. All of the following may contribute to sexual disinterest:

Biological factors: hormonal imbalance or insufficiencies, neurotransmitter imbalances, medications and their side effects, acute or chronic illnesses.

Developmental factors: lack of sexual education or permission; a childhood or adolescence marked by emotional, physical, verbal, or affectionate deprivation; sexual trauma or coercion.

Psychological factors: anxiety, depression, attachment disorders, personality or other psychiatric disorders.

Interpersonal factors: relationship discord, insults, losses, or partner sexual incompetence or dysfunction.

Cultural factors: religious or cultural mores and beliefs concerning appropriate sexual conduct.

Contextual factors: environmental factors such as privacy, safety, and comfort with surroundings.

Alternatively, desire problems are sometimes viewed as resulting from a variety of predisposing, precipitating, developmental, and maintaining factors (Althof et al., 2004):

Predisposing factors include constitutional attributes such as temperament (shyness vs. impulsivity, anatomical variations or deformities, inhibition vs. excitation, personality traits).

Developmental factors include problematical attachment experiences with parents, exposure to physical or sexual violence, negative early sexual experiences, and so forth.

Precipitating factors can include life-stage stressors such as divorce, infidelity, menopausal complaints, substance abuse, or humiliating or shameful experiences.

Maintaining factors may include ongoing stress, fatigue, relationship conflict, or body image concerns.

Given the heterogeneity of contributing factors, and the multiplicity of considerations that are relevant to both the initiation and the maintenance of sexual desire difficulties, the clinician must be creative and skillful in planning sensible and effective treatment. It is obvious that there can be no "one-size-fits all" model for therapeutic intervention. As will be evident from the clinical illustrations presented in this volume, each case is unique—every individual has an idiosyncratic erotic blueprint or love map that may complement or conflict with that of a partner. When erotic blueprints are in sync, couples easily negotiate small differences in desire. When they clash, desire problems may be more problematical to treat. And, from another perspective, it is worth noting, as David Schnarch suggests in Chapter 3, that low desire and high desire are often mutable positions in a relationship system. Furthermore, the low-desire individual in one relationship may be the high-desire partner in a new and different relationship.

PRIMARY VERSUS SECONDARY VERSUS SITUATIONAL DESIRE

In diagnosing sexual desire disorders, it is important to ascertain whether the complaint is primary or secondary, acute or chronic, and acquired or generalized. Acute and situational problems usually have a better prognosis than primary, generalized, and chronic lack of desire. While there are many factors that may contribute to a secondary loss of desire, the full range of possible components can be daunting. Such factors can span everything from transient partner conflict or the impact of disease or medication to a primary generalized lack of sexual interest, where there is a total absence of sexual fantasies or thoughts, masturbation, or any manifestation of sexual curiosity or arousal. While some authors in this volume do report success in treating such cases of primary absence (see Chapter 12, by Korda, Goldstein, and Goldstein), the majority of successful cases described in this book deal with situational or secondary lack of desire. In fact, many clinicians report frustration and failure in their attempts to generate sexual interest in cases where the individual reports a lifelong absence of desire.

DIAGNOSTIC ASSESSMENT:
INTERVIEW AND INSTRUMENTS

There are several standardized instruments and questionnaires for assessing desire complaints (see Table 1.1), but nothing really replaces the clinical interview where the individual and his or her partner are seen individually and as a couple. Much light can be shed by learning about the upbringing, family relationships, myths, and messages each partner brings to the relationship, as well as by observing the verbal and nonverbal exchanges of a couple together. Most of the chapters in this volume attest to the utility of interviewing and treating desire problems from a relational perspective.

PHARMACOTHERAPY FOR DESIRE DISORDERS

At this time, there are very few pharmacological interventions for enhancing desire. While sildenafil (Viagra) and the other phosphodiesterase (PD5) inhibitors (Levitra and Cialis) have proven extremely useful in treating male erectile dysfunction, they do little for increasing sexual desire itself in men (or women). One recent study did suggest that sildenafil was a helpful adjunct in women experiencing sexual dysfunction associated with antidepressant treatment (Nurnberg et al., 2008). One of the more prosexual antidepressants is bupropion (Wellbutrin), which has a lower incidence of sexual side effects than the selective serotonin reuptake inhibitor antidepressants. There is promising research under way with a new centrally acting drug, flibanserin, for the treatment of HSDD in premenopausal women, but as of this writing it is not FDA approved. In Chapter 13, Bonnie R. Saks provides a useful overview of the adjunctive use of medications in working with individuals with desire problems.

WHY THIS BOOK?

Desire complaints present a genuine conundrum. As we have seen, changes in the amount or intensity of sexual desire are normative and often inevitable over the course of a relationship, with life stresses and developmental milestones, hormonal changes, and medications. Nothing stays the same as we grow older and sexual desire is no exception. The problem is often with false expectations—with the fantasy that sexual desire is somehow immune from the whole array

TABLE 1.1. Scales for Assessing Desire/Arousal Problems

Assessment of sexual desire/arousal problems is critical in planning meaningful and sensible treatment interventions. The most common approach to diagnosing sexual difficulties is via a comprehensive clinical interview of both the identified patient and his or her partner. Such an interview includes discussion about the presenting problem and the predisposing, precipitating, and maintaining factors that govern its appearance and intensity (Grazziotin & Leiblum, 2005). It is also important to explore current contextual factors that affect sexual expression and interest, such as relationship satisfaction, privacy issues, current health of self and partner, medical or psychiatric issues, use of medications or recreational drugs/alcohol that may affect sexual expression, and current stressors.

Many clinicians find that the use of standardized self-report questionnaires can be helpful initially in terms of saving time, identifying problem areas, and providing direction or focus for a more extended clinical interview.

The following brief assessment tools have demonstrated good reliability and validity:

- *Brief Index of Sexual Functioning for Women* (Taylor, Rosen, & Leiblum, 1994). A 22-item questionnaire that provides domain and total scores on the following aspects of sexual function: desire, arousal, frequency of sexual activity, receptivity/initiation, pleasure/orgasm, relationship satisfaction, and problems affecting sexual function.

- *Decreased Sexual Desire Screener* (Clayton et al., 2009). An easy-to-use five-question instrument that provides rapid identification of generalized, acquired female hypoactive sexual desire. It consists of four yes/no questions to determine whether a desire problem and related distress exist. The more inclusive fifth question permits elaboration of possible contributing or maintaining factors.

- *Female Sexual Function Index* (Rosen et al., 2000). A 19-item questionnaire specific to women that assesses six domains (desire, subjective arousal, lubrication, orgasm, satisfaction, and pain). It has been widely used in outcome research and has good validity and reliability for diagnosing a variety of sexual complaints.

- *Female Sexual Distress Scale* (Derogatis et al., 2002). A 12-item assessment instrument used to determine the amount of current distress experienced by a woman with sexual difficulties. A cutoff score of 15 or greater is associated with personal distress.

- *Female Sexual Distress Scale—Revised* (Derogatis, 2008). The most recent validation of the Sexual Distress Scale, which was undertaken in order to enhance the sensitivity of the instrument for patients experiencing HSDD. The new question that was included is: "Are you bothered by low sexual desire?" and the respondent circles never (0), rarely (1), occasionally (2), frequently (3), or always (4).

- *Golombok–Rust Inventory of Sexual Satisfaction* (Rust & Golombok, 1986). A 28-item questionnaire that encompasses five domains relevant to women: anorgasmia, vaginismus, female avoidance, nonsensuality, and female dissatisfaction.

- *HSDD Screener* (Leiblum et al., 2006). A four-item screener that asks about loss of desire and distress in postmenopausal women.

- *Sexual Desire Inventory* (Spector, Carey, & Steinberg, 1996). A 14-item questionnaire that measures domains of dyadic and solitary sexual desire.

- *Sexual Function Questionnaire* (Quirk et al., 2002). A relatively new instrument designed to assess eight domains of women's sexuality: desire, physical arousal/sensation, physical arousal/lubrication, enjoyment, orgasm, pain, partner relationship, and cognition.

of changes that occur with aging, that while we may lose our hair and pack on the pounds, we somehow can maintain the sexual desire we had as 18-year-olds.

Ridiculous, we all agree. And yet, while lack of desire is not a life-threatening problem, it is often distressing and problematical to relationships and to our comfort with and satisfaction in them. A partner who is repeatedly sexually rejected or only reluctantly accepted feels hurt and frustrated and, finally, will often become angry or depressed. Over time, the sense of intimate connection with a partner is compromised. There is less physical teasing or affection, fewer spontaneous hugs or passionate kisses. Physical avoidance may replace affectionate snuggling since affection may be misinterpreted as a sexual invitation.

Alternatively, there may develop a greater reliance on pornography or masturbation. Often, there is the defensive decision on the part of the rejected partner that if any sexual intimacy is to occur, it must be initiated by the low-desire mate; the pain of rejection has become too great. The relationship is described as one of "roommates" rather than "lovers."

Whether seen as a psychiatric diagnosis or a relationship problem, complaints involving too little, too much, or discrepant desire are indeed legitimate concerns that warrant intervention. But how to intervene? Typically, desire concerns are not only frustrating to a client or couple, they are frustrating to the clinician as well. Anecdotally, many therapists say that they "dread" cases involving desire problems because they are uncertain about how to successfully intervene. There are no cookbooks or prescriptions for creating desire.

Clinicians also sometimes wonder if it is even *possible* to ignite desire where none has existed. Can the person who reports lifelong sexual apathy become sexually motivated or receptive? Should he or she be encouraged to? Can sex become lusty when it has become lackluster? What are reasonable expectations or treatment goals in these cases?

These are the questions that prompted this book. In order to find answers, prominent and expert clinicians of varying persuasions, training, and therapeutic philosophies were asked how they approach and treat desire problems. What has (or has not!) worked for these experienced and thoughtful clinicians?

Of course, given the complex and multifactorial etiology of desire complaints, there is not (and never will be) a standardized treatment. But seeing how top-notch therapists think about desire cases is illuminating. The contributors to this volume represent a wide spectrum of backgrounds and training. Each is skilled in his or her craft and has earned the title of expert. The chapters that follow are both provocative and stimulating. They challenge stereotypes and they reject the chimera of easy remedies for complex problems. But above all they constitute a thoughtful, nuanced, and pragmatic reflection of the many approaches to the assessment and treatment of desire complaints in current clinical practice.

This book does not attempt to be comprehensive in its overview. While there has been an attempt to balance examples involving men and women, gay and straight, older and younger clients, the authors were free to select cases they believed were representative of their clientele and treatment philosophy. It is to be hoped that the reader will come away from this volume with an increased appreciation of the spectrum of approaches and interventions for assisting individuals and couples with desire issues, and will feel awe and admiration for the artful interventions of these skilled clinicians.

REFERENCES

Althof, S., Leiblum, S., Chevert-Measson, M., Hartman, U., Levine, S., McCabe, M., et al. (2004). Psychological and interpersonal dimensions of sexual function and dysfunction. In T. Lue et al. (Eds.), *Sexual medicine: Sexual dysfunctions in men and women* (pp. 75–115). Paris: Second International Consultation on Sexual Dysfunctions.

American Psychiatric Association. (1980). *Diagnostic and statistical manual of mental disorders* (3rd ed.). Washington, DC: Author.

American Psychiatric Association. (1994). *Diagnostic and statistical manual of mental disorders* (4th ed.). Washington, DC: Author.

American Psychiatric Association. (2000). Diagnostic and statistical manual of mental disorders (4th ed., text rev.). Washington, DC: Author.

Basson, R. (2001). Using a different model for female sexual response to address women's problematic low desire. *Journal of Sex and Marital Therapy, 5*, 395–403.

Basson, R. (2002). Rethinking low sexual desire in women. *British Journal of Obstetrics and Gynecology, 4*, 357–363.

Basson, R., & Leiblum, S. (2003). Letter to the editor re: women's sexual dysfunction. *British Medical Journal, 326*(7390), 658.

Basson, R., Leiblum, S., Brotto, L., Derogatis, L., Fourcroy, J., Fugl-Meyer, K., et. al. (2003). Definitions of women's sexual dysfunctions reconsidered: Advocating expansion and revision. *Journal of Psychosomatic Obstetrics & Gynaecology, 24*, 221–229.

Beach, F. (1956). Characteristics of masculine "sex drive." In M. Jones (Ed.), *Nebraska Symposium on Motivation* (pp. 1–32). Lincoln: University of Nebraska Press.

Bergner, D. (2009, February 3). What do women want? *New York Times Magazine*. Available online *www.nytimes.com/2009/01/23/health/23iht-25desiret.19636765.html*.

Bogaert, A. F. (2004). Asexuality: Prevalence and associated factors in a national probability sample. *Journal of Sex Research, 41*(3), 279–287.

Bogaert, A. F. (2006). Toward a conceptual understanding of asexuality. *Review of General Psychology, 10*(3), 241–250.

Buster, J., Kingsberg, S., Aguirre, O., Brown, C., Wekselman, K., & Casso, P. (2004, June 16–19). *Large Phase III study confirms that transdermal testosterone patch 300 pg/day significantly improves sexual function with minimal side effects in surgically menopausal women*. Abstract presented at the annual meeting of the Endocrine Society, New Orleans, LA.

Chivers, M. (2005). A brief review and discussion of sex differences in the specificity of sexual arousal. *Sexual and Relationship Therapy, 20*, 377–390.

Chivers, M., Rieger, G., Latty, E., & Bailey, M. (2004). A sex difference in the specificity of sexual arousal. *Psychological Science, 15*, 736–744.

Clayton, A., Goldfischer, E., Goldstein, I., Derogatis, L., Lewis-D'Agostino, D., & Pyke, R. (2009). Validation of the decreased sexual desire screener (DSDS): A brief diagnostic instrument for generalized acquired female hypoactive sexual desire disorder (HSDD). *Journal of Sexual Medicine, 6*, 730–738.

Davis, S., Davison, S., Donath, S., & Bell, R. (2005). Circulating androgen levels and self-reported sexual function in women. *Journal of the American Medical Association, 294*(1), 91–96.

Deeks, A. A., & McCabe, M. P. (2001). Sexual function and the menopausal woman: The importance of age and partner's sexual functioning. *Journal of Sex Research, 38*, 219–225.

Derogatis, L. (2008). Validation of the Female Sexual Distress Scale—Revised for assessing distress in women with hypoactive sexual desire disorder. *Journal of Sexual Medicine, 5*, 357–364.

Derogatis, L., Rosen, R., Leiblum, S., Burnett, A., & Heiman, J. (2002). The Female Sexual Distress Scale (FSDS): Initial validation of a standardized scale for assessment of sexually related personal distress in women. *Journal of Sex and Marital Therapy, 28*, 317–330.

Diamond, L. (2005). What we got wrong about sexual identity development: Unexpected findings from a longitudinal study of young women. In A. Omoto & H. Kurtzman (Eds.), *Sexual orientation and mental health: Examining identity and development in lesbian, gay, and bisexual people* (pp. 73–94). Washington, DC: American Psychological Association.

Freud, S. (1962). *Three essays on the theory of sexuality*. New York: Avon Books. (Original work published 1905)

Graziottin, A., & Leiblum, S. (2005). Biological and psychosocial pathophysiology of female sexual dysfunction during the menopausal transition. *Journal of Sexual Medicine*, Suppl. 3, 133–145.

Hayes, R., Bennett, C., Fairle, C., & Dennerstein, L. (2006). What can prevalence studies tell us about female sexual difficulty or dysfunction? *Journal of Sexual Medicine*, 3, 589–595.

Hayes, R., Dennerstein, L., Bennett, C., & Fairley, C. (2008). What is the "true" prevalence of female sexual dysfunctions and does the way we assess these conditions have an impact? *Journal of Sexual Medicine*, 5, 777–787.

Hayes, R. D., Dennerstein, L., Bennett, C. M., Koochaki, P. E., Leiblum, S. R., & Graziottin, A. (2007). Relationship between hypoactive sexual desire disorder and aging. *Fertility and Sterility*, 87, 107–112.

Johnson, M. T. (1977). Asexual and autoerotic women: Two invisible groups. H. L. Gochros & J. S. Gochros (Eds.), *The sexually oppressed* (pp. 96–109). New York: Associated Press.

Kaplan, H. (1977). Hypoactive sexual desire. *Journal of Sex and Marital Therapy*, 3, 3–9.

Laumann, E., Gagnon, J., Michael, R., & Michaels, S. (1994). *The social organization of sexuality: Sexual practices in the United States*. Chicago: University of Chicago Press.

Leiblum, S. R., & Rosen, R. C. (1988). Introduction: Changing perspectives on sexual desire. In S. R. Leiblum & R. C. Rosen (Eds.), *Sexual desire disorders* (pp. 1–17). New York: Guilford Press.

Leiblum, S. R., Symonds, T., Moore, J., Soni, P., Steinberg, S., & Sisson, M. (2006). A methodology study to develop and validate a screener for hypoactive sexual desire disorder in postmenopausal women. *Journal of Sexual Medicine*, 3, 455–464.

Lief, H. (1977). Inhibited sexual desire. *Medical Aspects of Human Sexuality*, 7, 94–95.

Maurice, W. L. (2007). Sexual desire disorders in men. In S. R. Leiblum (Ed.), *Principles and practice of sex therapy* (4th ed., pp. 181–211). New York: Guilford Press.

McKinlay, J., & Feldman, H. (1994). Age-related variation in sexual activity and interest in normal men: Results from the Massachusetts Male Aging Study. In A. S. Rossi (Ed.), *Sexuality across the life course* (pp. 261–285). Chicago: University of Chicago Press.

Mercer, C., Fenton, K., Johnson, A., Wellings, K., Macdowall, W., McManus, S., et al. (2003). Sexual function problems and help seeking behaviors in Britain: National probability sample survey. *British Medical Journal*, 327, 426–427.

Meston, C., & Buss, D. (2007). Why humans have sex. *Archives of Sexual Behavior*, 36(4), 477–507.

Moynihan, R. (2003). The making of a disease: Female sexual dysfunction. *British Medical Journal, 326,* 45–47.

Nurnberg, H., Hensley, P., Heiman, J., Croft, H., Debattista, C., & Paine, S. (2008). Sildenafil treatment of women with antidepressant-associated sexual dysfunction: A randomized controlled trial. *Journal of the American Medical Association, 300*(4), 395–404.

Quirk, F. H., Heiman, J. R., Rosen, R. C., Laan, E., Smith, M. D., & Boolell, M. (2002). Development of a Sexual Function Questionnaire for Clinical Trials of Female Sexual Dysfunction. *Journal of Women's Health and Gender-Based Medicine, 11*(3), 277–289.

Richters, J., Grulich, A. E., de Visser, R. O., Smith, A. M. A., & Rissel, C. E. (2001). Sex in Australia: Sexual difficulties in a representative sample of adults. *Australian and New Zealand Journal of Public Health, 27,* 164–170.

Rosen, R., Brown, C., Heiman, J., Leiblum, S., Meston, C., Shabsigh, R., et al. (2000). The Female Sexual Function Index (FSFI): A multidimensional self-report instrument for the assessment of female sexual function. *Journal of Sex and Marital Therapy, 26,* 191–208.

Rust, J., & Golombok, S. (1986). The GRISS: A psychometric instrument for the assessment of sexual dysfunction. *Archives of Sexual Behavior, 15,* 157–165.

Schneidewind-Skibbe, A., Hayes, R., Koochaki, P., Meyer, J., & Dennerstein, L. (2008). The frequency of sexual intercourse reported by women: A review of community-based studies and factors limiting their conclusions. *Journal of Sexual Medicine, 5,* 301–335.

Shifren, J., Davis, S., Moreau, M., Waldbaum, A., Bouchard, C. D., DeRogatis, L., et. al. (2006). Testosterone path for the treatment of hypoactive sexual desire disorder in naturally menopausal women: Results from the INTIMATE NM1 Study. *Menopause, 13*(5), 770–779.

Simon, J., Braunstein, G., Nachtigall, L., Utian, W., Katz, M., Miller, S., et al. (2005). Testosterone patch increases sexual activity and desire in surgically menopausal women with hypoactive sexual desire disorder. *Journal of Clinical Endocrinology and Metabolism, 90*(9), 5226–5233.

Simon, J., Nachtigall, L., Davis, S., Utian, W., Lucas, J., & Braunstein, G. (2004). Transdermal testosterone patch improves sexual activity and desire in surgically menopausal women. *Obstetrics & Gynecology, 103*(Suppl. 4), 64S.

Spector, I., Carey, M., & Steinberg, L. (1996). The sexual desire inventory: Development, factor structure, and evidence of reliability. *Journal of Sex and Marital Therapy, 22,* 175–190.

Taylor, J., Rosen, R., & Leiblum, S. (1994). Self-report assessment of female sexual function: Psychometric evaluation of the brief index of sexual functioning for women. *Archives of Sexual Behavior, 23*(6), 627–643.

Wang, C., Nieschlag, E., Swerdloff, R., Behre, H., Hellstrom, W., Gooren, L., et al. (2009). ISA, ISSAM, EAU, EAA and ASA recommendations:

Investigation, treatment and monitoring of late-onset hypogonadism in males. *International Journal of Impotence Research, 21*(1), 1–8.

Weijmar Schultz, W. C. M., & Van de Wiel, H. (1991). Sexual functioning after gyneacecological cancer treatment. Unpublished doctoral dissertation, Rijksuniversiteit Groningen, the Netherlands.

Weijmar Schultz, W. C. M., & Van de Wiel, H. B. M. (2003). Sexuality, intimacy, and gynecological cancer. *Journal of Sex and Marital Therapy, 29*, 121–128.

Whalen, R. (1966). Sexual motivation. *Psychological Review, 73*, 151–163.

Chapter 2

The Double Flame

Reconciling Intimacy and Sexuality, Reviving Desire

Esther Perel

"Love is about having and desire is about wanting." This is the major observation that guides Esther Perel's therapy as she works with couples complaining of loss of desire. She observes that lack of desire does not necessarily reflect a disordered relationship and that erotic ruts are part of being a loving, caring couple. She lays out a paradox: the very ingredients that nurture love are often the ones that erode erotic passion. Perel turns the usual therapeutic approach on its head with this suggestion: first improve the sex, an improved relationship will follow.

In order to reconcile the paradox that inevitably exists between the wish for an all-knowing intimacy and the heightened passion that accompanies the unfamiliar and unpredictable, it is necessary to cultivate mystery and tolerate separation. As she observes, "Desire balks at consistency and is motored by absence and longing." Fantasy and imagination constitute key ingredients in liberating and reawakening desire, not insistence, demands, or negotiation. It is not the innovative techniques she is after, but the experience of anticipation surrounding the mystery of the other and the unknown in ourselves.

In her fascinating case description, Perel illustrates how the unique erotic blueprints of Alicia and Roberto developed and were initially effective in supporting their erotic life. But in their current relationship they have fallen into the familiar roles of pursuer and distancer, which satisfies neither. Furthermore, the way they are emotionally organized around each other is too reminiscent of their original families, which inevitably numbs all forms of sexual expressiveness.

The therapy engages the partners to uncover and to free themselves from their erotic blocks. Like so many women, Alicia dislikes Roberto's sexual directness, which she experiences as neediness. She wants seduction and transgression to lift her from her internalized prohibitions. For Roberto, familiarity breeds content and he values comfort and intimacy to spark his desire. Once they are encouraged to use their imagination and to discover new ways of seducing and beguiling each other, their erotic desire increases.

Perel concludes her chapter with the reminder that in long-term relationships, active engagement and willful intent are needed to nurture eroticism and maintain desire.

Esther Perel, MA, LMFT, is a practicing marital and family therapist in New York City. She is the author of *Mating in Captivity: Reconciling the Erotic and the Domestic*, which has been translated into 24 languages. She is recognized as one of the most original and provocative theorists in the field of sex therapy today.

THE DOMESTIC AND THE EROTIC

As a couple therapist, I see young and old, married or not, gay, bisexual, and straight, with passports from all over the world. Plenty has changed in my 25 years of private practice, but not my patients' opening lines. They tend to go something like this: "We love each other very much, but we have no sex." Next they'll move into describing relationships that are open and loving, yet sexually dull. Time and again they tell me of the paradoxical relationship between domesticity and sexual desire. They treasure the stability, security, and predictability of a committed relationship, they miss the excitement, novelty, and mystery that eroticism thrives on.

When they complain about the listlessness of their sex lives, they sometimes want more frequent sex, but they always want "better" sex. They want to recapture the feeling of connection, playfulness, and renewal that sex used to allow them.

Modern committed couples have a long list of sexual alibis that claim to explain the death of eros. They are too busy, too stressed, and too tired for sex. Eventually lamentations about the kids, the house, the job trail off, and more complex and nuanced obstacles come forward: couples who are such good friends they cannot sustain being lovers; lovers so set on spontaneity that sex never happens at all. I see power struggles that escalate into erotic stalemates, emotional arrangements that are overly familial and blatantly desexualizing. Some clients feel sheepish, others rejected, and some are just plain confused—all of them, however, have experienced a genuine loss.

So why does great sex so often fade for couples who love each other as much as ever? Why does good intimacy not guarantee good sex? Why does the transition to parenthood spell erotic disaster? Can we want what we already have? Why is the forbidden so erotic? When we love, how does it feel, and when we desire, how is it different?

I seek to probe the ambiguities of love and desire in long-term relations, to explore the fears and anxieties that arise when our pursuit of safety and security clashes with our quest for passion and adventure. We seek predictability on one hand, and thrive on discovery and adventure on the other. Psychoanalyst Steven A. Mitchell (2002) makes the point that these are two fundamental, yet opposing human needs that pull us in different directions. Partners today need to negotiate their dual needs for *familiarity and novelty*, their wish for *certainty and surprise*. Yet it is difficult to generate excitement and anticipation with the same person we look to for comfort and stability.

In the West we take for granted the idea that marriage is the key to everything. We turn to one person to fulfill what an entire village (friends, community, extended family) once delivered. We expect our partners to be the primary supplier for our emotional connections, to provide the anchoring experiences of life. Intimacy and transparency in the romantic marriage are paramount, meant to help us transcend the aloneness of modern existence and be a bulwark against the vicissitudes of everyday life. We seek security, as we always have, but now we also want our partner to love us, cherish us, and excite us. For the first time in history, we have sex not because we want eight kids or because it's the woman's marital duty; today's couples count on desire and sexual fulfillment as key ingredients to a happy marriage. I believe we must recognize that reconciling the erotic and the domestic is not a problem we can solve, it is a paradox we manage.

THE NUMBING OF DESIRE

Traditional couple therapy believes that sexual problems stem from relationship problems. Poor communication, lack of intimacy, and accumulated resentments are some of the explanations given to explain the numbing of desire. Find out about the state of the union first, see how it manifests in the bedroom second. The premise is that a troubled relationship equals no sex; improve the emotional relationship, and the desire will follow.

But my practice suggests otherwise. I've helped plenty of couples buff up their relationship and it did nothing for the sex. It made a difference in the kitchen, but it did little for the bedroom. Strengthening the caring and the companionate affection is often not enough to generate erotic desire. In such situations, I invert the traditional therapeutic priorities, asking about the partners' sexuality first. It becomes a window into the self, the couple's dynamics, and their families of origin. I flip the equation: improve the sex, and the relationship will follow. Sex is not a metaphor for the relationship, but rather a parallel narrative, one that speaks its own language.

Love and desire—they relate and they conflict, and herein lies the mystery of eroticism. The rules of desire are not the same as the rules of good citizenship. It is not always the lack of closeness that stifles desire, but too much closeness. Many couples are disappointed to discover that the closeness and comfort they crave are exactly what douses the fire. More intimacy doesn't always make for more sex. In fact, sometimes the very qualities that nurture intimacy—grounding, familiarity, and continuity—can be sexually deflating and drain the passion right out of our relationships.

Stability, understanding, and compassion are the handmaidens of a close, harmonious relationship, while eroticism thrives on novelty, mystery, and the unexpected. There is a complex relationship between love and desire—between a couple's emotional life together and their physical life together, and these don't always correspond. What is emotionally satisfying isn't necessarily sexually exciting. That's one reason why, to the chagrin of many, you can often "fix" the relationship and it will not do anything for the sex. Intimacy begets sexuality only sometimes.

If love is about having, desire is about wanting. Love wants to contract distance, and minimize the threat; it wants to collapse the tension. It seeks closeness and wants to know the beloved. Desire balks at consistency and is motored by absence and longing. For some of us, love and desire are inseparable. But for many others, emotional intimacy inhibits erotic expression. For them, the caring, protective elements that foster love block the freedom and unself-consciousness that fuel erotic pleasure.

Let me illustrate: Think of a little child who sits comfortably nestled on your lap. At some point she jumps off and runs out. At a distance, she stops, turns, and get her cues from the adult she just left. If the adult says, "Go ahead, kiddo, the world is a beautiful place with lots to discover. Have fun," the little child turns away and runs further. She experiences both freedom and connection, and at the same time, the security of love and the autonomy of desire. This child who plays hide and seek will one day turn to eroticism as the adult version of hide and seek, where she'll maintain playfulness and discovery, alternating between the dangers of hiding and seeking and the relief of finding and being found.

There is, however, another scenario with a very different outcome. This time the adult says: "What's so beautiful out there? Isn't being together enough? I am lonely, I am anxious, depressed … " Here, the child has a few choices. One of them is to return to base. They learn that in order not to lose that connection with the other, they'll have to lose a part of themselves. In my experience these are often the people who, later on, will have a hard time making love to the person they love. The legacy of this bargain for attachment produces a puzzling inverse correlation where growing intimacy leads to diminished desire. In his book *Arousal: The Secret Logic of Sexual Fantasies*, Michael Bader (2002) explains that it isn't a fear of intimacy or a lack of commitment that solders their block, rather it is the nature of their love—burdensome and confining—that stands in the way of the desire. The worry and responsibility they feel for their beloved forecloses the necessary spontaneity and selfishness for erotic abandon.

Sexual intimacy is an act of generosity and self-centeredness, of giving and taking. We need to be able to enter another without the terror that we will be swallowed and lose ourselves. At the same time we need to be able to enter ourselves, to surrender to self-absorption while in the presence of the other, believing that they will still be there when we return, that they won't feel rejected by our momentary absence. The self absorption inherent in sexual excitement obliterates the other in a way that collides with the ideal of intimacy. So many people believe that they can be safely lustful and intemperate only with people they don't know as well, or care about as much.

Tell me how you were loved, I'll tell you how you make love. This is a construct I often work with. Our sexual preferences arise from the thrills, challenges, and conflicts of our early life. How these bear on our threshold for closeness and pleasure is the object of our excavation. Not coincidentally, our entire emotional history plays itself out in the physicality of sex, and our erotic blueprints are layered with these childhood experiences.

FIRE NEEDS AIR

Desire wants to go where it hasn't yet been. It needs otherness, difference. But for erotic élan there needs to be a synapse to cross. Modern couples strive for oneness, yet eroticism thrives in the space between self and the other.

Because this concept may seem abstract, I routinely ask the following question: "When do you feel most drawn, most attracted to your partner?" The answers resonate with a remarkable similarity.

> "After we've been apart ..., when he's confident and passionate about something he loves.... When she's unaware I'm watching her.... When he is talking with friends.... When he surprises me.... When we're at a party and I see others looking at her.... When she's standing on the other side of a crowded room, and she smiles just for me.... When he's playing with the kids.... [This is the only comment that is gender specific, for men rarely think that a mother playing with the kids is sexy.] When we're away from home, and have fun together.... When we dance ... When I ride on the back of his motorcycle ... When I see him play sports...."

Whatever the answer, it is never without an element of distance. It is a description where we look at our partner from a comfortable distance. Not too close because we cannot distinguish them from ourselves, and not too far, for then they are no longer in our field of vision. We see a partner who is separate, whose difference is magnified. And this person who is otherwise already so familiar is momentarily once again somewhat unknown, somewhat mysterious and elusive. More importantly, in none of these situations is the other needing us, nor do we need to take care of him or her. Caretaking may be very loving, but it is also a powerful anti-aphrodisiac. In sex, people want to feel wanted, not needed.

We create a bridge of things unknown by making a perceptual shift, and it is on this bridge, in the space *between* us, that we can meet and play with the erotic. Sometimes introducing mystery is nothing more than a shift in perception. In the words of Proust, "The real voyage of discovery consists not in seeking new landscapes but in having new eyes."

The question posed earlier—"Can we want what we already have?"—invites us to admit that we never "have" our partners. It is our willingness to engage with the mystery that keeps desire alive. Faced with the irrefutable otherness of our partner, we can respond with fear or with curiosity. We can try to reduce them to a knowable entity, or we can embrace their persistent mystery. When we resist the urge to control, when we keep ourselves open, we preserve the possibility of discovery. Eroticism resides in the ambiguous space between anxiety and fascination. We remain interested in our partners; they delight us, and we're drawn to them. It is not mere emotional anxiety, but rather the existential reality that there is no permanence, no lasting holding. When we trade passion for reality, maybe we are just trading one fiction for another. In the words of therapist Anthony Robbins, passion is commensurate with the amount of uncertainty we can tolerate.

EROTICISM AS ALIVENESS, PLEASURE, IMAGINATION

My interest is in the erotic, not only in the act of sex. The physical act of sex is often too narrow and it easily degenerates into conversations about numbers and performance. The erotic landscape is vastly larger, richer, and more intricate than the physiology of sex or any repertoire of sexual techniques. What people long for is radiance, beating back deadness.

This focus on eroticism comes from my work with traumatized populations and from growing up in a community of Holocaust survivors, where I always observed two groups. There were those who did not die, and those who came back to live. Those who didn't die lived quite tethered to the ground, pouring their energies into finding basic trust, alleviating their fears, and guarding against a dangerous world outside. Pleasure for them was fraught with guilt and fear. Those who came back to live were eager to reenter the world, forge ahead, reconnect with playfulness and pleasure and take risks. They understood how to cultivate aliveness, vibrancy; they experienced the erotic as an antidote to death. This distinction also applies to the couples I work with: there are those who survive and those who are alive. I think of eroticism beyond the sexual meaning that modernity has assigned to it. Couples who have an erotic spark know how to cultivate a sense of aliveness, vibrancy, and vitality over the long haul. They understand that the central agent of eroticism is the imagination. Not the one that focuses on new sexual positions, but one where we continue to imagine our partner with a compelling curiosity and we remain interesting and attractive to ourselves.

SEX AND INTIMACY SPEAK MANY LANGUAGES

No matter which country you are from, which language you first spoke, it is the language of the body that is the universal mother tongue. The body is a vital language, a conduit for emotional intimacy. As Roland Barthes wrote, "What language conceals is said through my body. My body is a stubborn child, my language is a very civilized adult."

The modern world of coupledom has done much in the way of censoring both men and women in this primal parlance. For men, the body is often the center of tenderness and vulnerability, and it longs to speak. Our emphasis (or overemphasis, rather) on the macho, power-driven aspects of male sexuality works to mute the very expression we seek. Conversely, for women, the emphasis is on words, estranging them from a rich panoply of connection to their bodies. Any thoughts of lustfulness, physicality, or hunger are legitimized only when layered in relatedness or duty. With sex and intimacy at the epicenter of the couple's identity, they need to give themselves permission to be bilingual.

In the case example that follows, I illustrate how these concepts play out and how I use them to reignite desire in a couple that have lost their erotic life.

CASE EXAMPLE: ALICIA AND ROBERTO

Alicia and Roberto, an attractive, intelligent, and loving couple come for treatment, complaining of their moribund sex life. Alicia is 30, born in a small village in Andalucia, to a devout Catholic bourgeois family. Her mother came from a family of 12 children, ruled under the strict authority of her father. After meeting her husband-to-be she married him quickly and was whisked away. They both shared the impatience of those who can't wait to leave the hamlet and migrate to the big city, get an education, and move abroad. This is exactly what they did, with two daughters in tow. Alicia was the oldest, and in her words: "I was my mom's object."

In the various European countries where her family lived, she could attend local schools but not become a local girl. Her mother was critical of the permissiveness she saw in the postmodern families. Like many other traditional immigrant families who confront today's Western culture of family democracy and its unprecedented child centrality, Alicia's parents were critical of the permissiveness they observed. They feared that unregulated freedom would expose their daughters to male predators, who would take advantage of them, sexually and emotionally.

Mom and Dad divorced, and the restrictions only grew. Alicia had to jump through the window to play with her friends and rendezvous with her secret boyfriend. She pieced together a sexual education bit by bit. From Mom she learned about the birds and the bees and menstruation, and received warnings about sexual dangers. From her friends she picked up her knowledge of romance and fun. One day she was caught and severely punished for being with her boyfriend. She opted for depression rather than rebellion.

With Alicia in a state of despondence, and Grandpa, the patriarch, dead, her mother started therapy. Surprisingly, she embarked on a systematic journey of rejection and transformation. Once a traditional, religious, compliant, rule-based, sexually numb, and discipline-driven woman, she became independent, pleasure seeking, emancipated, and liberated. She transformed so much that, according to Alicia, she jumped two centuries in 2 years.

Roberto's roots were Andalucian as well. His grandfather was a world traveler, who brought his bewitching, dark-eyed Mediterranean woman to the Americas. At 33, Roberto was about to start a degree in public policy. He described an affectionate family—a father who took him on long walks, where they enjoyed solving the riddles of the cosmos. Mom was a jewelry maker, caring but withdrawn, and hard to talk with. One day, Roberto confronted her about her hermetic character, and her response came with tears: "That's the way I am, I will not change." That was his last attempt to get through.

As far as he can remember, Roberto's parents never shared a bedroom, and only years later was he told why. Dad was physically and romantically effusive, Mom was not. So he took his hands and body to many other women. It was only in college that Roberto learned of the incessant dalliances of his father, a piece of information that became central to Roberto's life. For reasons he is only now starting to understand, he became a consummate lover. "Growing up, sex was a normal part of development. I didn't associate much anxiety with sex. It was a source of pleasure, a conduit for intimacy and bonding. When my mother found condoms in my room, she said it was smart that I was using protection."

Roberto liked girls, and girls liked him. He sampled and explored, and beginning with his first girlfriend, "I was purposeful and unfaithful. I became greedy, courting disaster to see how much I could handle at once without imploding. I was profoundly selfish, even though I was generous in bed. I was a master liar and cheater. Seeing how easy it was to lie, I became terrified it could be done to me." His jealousy on constant alert, Roberto was afraid to be deceived himself.

After college, Roberto traveled to Spain for a fellowship, ready for new emotional incursions. He met Alicia in Barcelona, where she was studying at the university. She took him by the hand, leading him through the winding narrow streets, and introduced him to her favorite tapas, and they got tipsy on sangria. They fell madly in love. Alicia was very different from his mother or other girlfriends—she was vivacious, outspoken, and exuberant. Their sex was fast-paced and adventurous. After a few months, they began a long-distance relationship that lasted almost 2 years. Technology was their trusted accomplice. Phone sessions, Skype sex, e-mails, texting, and a trip here and there added fuel to the flame.

Finally, Alicia moved to Philadelphia, joining Roberto in his tiny studio. The next phase of their relationship began. Immigration came with many demands—learning to speak English, acquiring a visa, finding a job. In addition, there was homesickness and the stress of living in a noisy city. Roberto tried to cushion the shock. He showed Alicia the ropes, wrote her application letters, and served as her cultural translator.

Within a few months, their sexual ardor declined and slowly faded away. They attributed it to the changes they were going through. As Roberto later tells me, "It made sense, but none of the explanations made a difference." Nevertheless, he wanted to make Alicia feel safe, so he curtailed his hobbies and social activities. Anything that Alicia didn't share with him was taken off the list, and with it, his individuality. While this made Alicia feel safe, it made Roberto feel suffocated. But he was fearful of making Alicia unhappy. After all, she had left friends and family in Spain for him. How could he ask for more? But without a sex life, he felt barren.

Roberto had always enjoyed a robust appetite for the pleasures of the flesh. For him, the plummeting of their sexual relation feels unending. He is frustrated and alarmed by the thought that things will never change and that he will revert to old behaviors of finding other women, but he is definite about one thing: he won't accept a carbon copy of his parents' relationship—a sexless marriage with a life of never-ending infidelities.

Initial Session

When I first meet the couple, they have been together for 6 years, the last 3 teetering on the verge of sexual collapse. Alicia is the one who withholds sexually, but she doesn't like the situation any more than Roberto. She vacillates between guilt and resentment, wishing he would not give up, and then demanding that he stop badgering her and leave her alone.

Roberto has become more clumsy, desperate, and unattractive. Alicia says she likes a confident man, but Roberto objects that it is difficult to remain confident in the face of constant criticism and rejection. More rejection leads to more loss of confidence, which leads to more neediness and then again more refusal.

Together we map the pattern of negative escalation, how it follows a sequence of complementary reactions. We draw from the other behaviors that match our expectations of them. The more Alicia reacts, the more Roberto pressures. The more he pressures, the more she distances, bemoaning his lack of subtlety. His desperate groping will make Alicia pull back even more although this is the opposite of what he wants. Her keeping him at bay will make him become even more needy, even though this is the last thing she wants. This dance of pursuit and distance is quite common, and on the surface it looks like a discrepancy of desire. I reflect that although it appears that Roberto wants sex and Alicia does not, in fact, they both are frustrated.

I know that Alicia is baffled by her lack of wanting. This is not the person she wants to be, nor the one she used to be and liked. As is often the case when people are mired in this predicament, when I ask Alicia to tell me about her sexual thoughts, she tells me about his. Her mind is filled with Roberto's wishes and disappointments, and she ends up being out of touch with her own wanting and feelings. Acutely aware of what *he* wants, she no longer knows what *she* wants.

I ask that she carry a notebook where she will write any erotic musings—catch them, write them, own them. We play with this tripartite equation, and in the coming weeks she will report if she was aware of having any sensations, feelings, thoughts, inclinations. At the next level, she'll see if she was able to bring them inside her: when we write, we commit ourselves on paper. And lastly, if she could own and remember them, it would help draw a boundary between her and Roberto, demarcating her sexual territory from his. This mindful exercise has been valuable and Alicia has been doing it since treatment began. Roberto is encouraged to do this as well.

In my work, I see the couple together, as well as individually. At times Alicia talks about her sexual meanderings alone, other times she shares them with Roberto. The individual sessions are always confidential. This allows each person to think alone, examine and clarify for themselves from a less defensive stance. They can decide what insights and questions they want to bring to the joint session, and how.

I see Alicia's block, but I don't immediately attribute it to a total lack of desire. I check: It is completely gone? On hold? Directed somewhere else? Alicia's sentence starts with "I have no desire," and I want to find out if the second part of the sentence will be "at home," "with him," or generally?

Our conversation veers to Alicia's dislike of Roberto's straightforwardness, his lack of suggestiveness, and blatant advances. "When he says, 'here's my cock, wanna take it' that is not playful for me. It's very American this pragmatic approach to sex," she says: "Direct, to the point, don't beat around the bush." "Does it diminish Roberto's sexual appeal?" I ask. She nods. Alicia taps into a common myth, the logic of which says: if I have to tell him what I like, what I am and what I want, it means he needs instructions, and if so, then he lacks intuitiveness, savoir faire. Conclusion: he is certainly not sexy, since a sexy man needs no tutorial.

At this time we unpack another cultural quandary. Historically and traditionally, the man who is sexually served by his wife needs no instructions, for what she wants is unimportant. But the man who hits the "right spots," the one who knows intuitively what she likes, is heralded as the man with the special touch, the one who doesn't need directions. Male arrogance has historically been met with female deference. But these stances continue to be reinforced today. While Alicia resents male superiority, she has difficulty accommodating to the alternative. When Roberto asks her for guidance, she regards him as less masculine. If he forges ahead with his lust, she reacts negatively about his lack of sensitivity.

Dismantling traditional gender roles takes a bit of psychological sleuthing, but little in one's erotic imagination is happenstance.

Alicia wants more play, not foreplay, an elaborate seduction, the "Juego," as she calls it—a choreography of seduction that alternates between approach and retreat, meant to stoke the wanting. The subtext reads: "You think I am attracted to you and that you can just have me, but you're wrong. You don't have me yet. Now I distance myself, I'll make you want me more. I come closer again and you think, this time, I got her. You're wrong again. I move away once more. You come after me. The more persistently you pursue me, the more attractive and irresistible I feel, which makes me move away some more to see if you'll keep coming after me, if I can make you want me even more."

Alicia tries to explain to Roberto that sex isn't something that starts at 7:00 and ends at 8:00. It's an attitude. Roberto replies that in the beginning Alicia didn't need any of this. She too was direct, aggressive, and open to the raw edge of desire. She recognizes his description, but she's in a different place now. Roberto is very open and willing—"I'll try anything." But rather than being receptive to Roberto's openness, Alicia responds that she doesn't like having to explain what she wants. I clarify that seduction isn't only about flooding the other with your wanting, but rather eliciting their own wanting—to seduce is not to induce. Roberto is willing to venture outside his comfort zone, but Alicia needs to be responsive. When she redirects his advances, she has to curb her criticisms. She can guide him and then resent him for not knowing, or she can appreciate a new generation of men who invite being directed and don't pretend to know.

I discuss with them that this playful attitude, the "Juego," is a way of relating to each other that is not just about being turned on, it is about maintaining an erotic interest for the other. They agree. I know that Alicia and Roberto play, but they describe it as "silly play," and while it's wonderful, it isn't sexy. It is a kind of play that is reminiscent of how children play: it can be sweet and affectionate, but it is unerotic. In fact, it often operates as a sexual appetite suppressor. When a couple becomes too familial, they desexualize the relationship. A hint of incestuousness hovers over them. Alicia points out that in order to engage in that *other* kind of play, she needs to feel safe; she is not interested in having that kind of play with a random person on the street. She'd like to be able to relax and let that side of her go, with him.

Roberto is intrigued by the fact that on one hand Alicia talks about wanting to be intimate with the person with whom she is playing these seductive games, but on the other hand, her predilection is for erotic games of anonymity, of not knowing the person. I clarify that play involving anonymity and fantasies about strangers—like going up to him at the gym and pretending she's never met him in the context of an intimate relationship—springs from a familiarity that's already been established. The secure connection is the base from which we freely enjoy "a room of one's own," and one for our partner as well.

Roberto tells me that for him, familiarity makes for better sex— he likes to feel comfortable, unencumbered. He likes the comfort released by emotional intimacy, the context, the sexual communication between him and his partner, and the ease he feels with himself. Comfortable is an erotic proposition for Roberto. When you feel familiar with someone, you no longer need to seduce, and the ease comes from the fact that the other person is there. At the same time, he's beginning to recognize that within this comfort, maybe he has not left enough space for himself, and that his striving for transparency and wholesale sharing isn't conducive to the mystery and the unknown that ignite desire.

For Alicia, "comfortable" resonates with "obvious" and with old expectations. "You're supposed to have sex with your husband, obviously," she says in her melodic Castilian accent. "And if it's what you should do?" I ask her. "Then it's not exciting," she replies. "Does obviousness stir rebelliousness?" I pursue. "Yes," she asserts. "When you emit a resounding no, you're certain not to do what you're supposed to do. It is a way to engage your free will." As things stand now, her sexual autonomy manifests as a sexual lobotomy.

Alicia makes the connection that coming from a strict Catholic rule-based upbringing she learned that sex was a duty performed by women for men. Roberto is quick to inquire, if he didn't want to have sex with her, would she be more interested? And the answer is yes, because it would release her from a feeling of duty and obligation and it would make room for her own independent wanting. It is difficult for her to want what he wants and still feel that it's her own. So if he were not interested, then she could come forward, and there would be a boundary delineating her interest. I clarify that Alicia's reaction isn't about him. It is about insubordination and autonomy, a rebellion against the confines of matrimony and the traditional role of women performing sexual duties.

There is another transaction between them that goes in the same direction. Alicia is often interested in sex with Roberto after they've had a fight—something that goes against everything he likes about the comfort and ease of sex. For Roberto, who is always ready for sex, this is the one time where he's really turned off. When he's angry he's less in touch with how much he cares for her. Fighting and arguments create a greater separateness. Fighting legitimizes our thoughts, our feelings, and our needs. When we defend our cause, we boost our sense of entitlement. After a fight Alicia's sense of obligation is lessened and her sense of autonomy is heightened. Hence, she can experience the freedom and the selfishness needed for desire while for Roberto the opposite is true.

Understanding our erotic blueprint involves tracing the cultural and familial messages that we were raised with. In Alicia's case, they were presented to her in black and white: premarital sex is forbidden, marital sex is for babies—a woman's duty toward her husband—and pleasure is sinful. And while rationally she no longer believes this, she feels that these beliefs are engraved inside of her, reinforced by her large family of 12 uncles and aunts. It appears that while mother and sister forged ahead on the new road, Alicia became the repository of all that had been left behind. "I am the one carrying our legacy. It's as if all the prohibitions of my Catholic upbringing have been transferred onto me. I'm the one who's caught in this sexual and emotional conundrum. It's as if it all stayed with me, all the taboos."

I am aware that the forbidden can be very erotic, and that transgression can be an essential ingredient, and so I ask Alicia, "If pleasure is sinful, how does the forbidden become pleasurable?" The anonymity of the back of the taxi, the public places, the restaurants—all those forbidden places invite a lustful transgression for her. Digging into the secret logic of sexual fantasies, Michael Bader (2002) explains that in the sanctuary of the erotic mind we find a psychological safe space to undo the inhibitions and fears that roil within us. Alicia's fantasies state the problems and offer the solution. Her sexual imagination allows her to negate and undo the limits imposed on her by her conscience, by her culture, and by her self-image. Simply put: If she doesn't know him, she is free of the traditional female sexual duty and obligation.

And with this new insight, Roberto is beginning to find his way through the maze of Alicia's erotic mind. At this point however, he needs reassurance. He worries that he would have to give up one type of closeness for another, that he would need to let go of a certain emotional intimacy in order to experience a sexual intimacy.

But Alicia doesn't make it easy for him. She feels she's at an impasse. She tells him of her conflict, between her love for the family she could have with him and the fact that family is the last place she can imagine having pleasurable sex. I suggest that they become cultural translators for one another and help each other navigate the split. I explain to them that I can imagine that all these public places, where you're not supposed to have sex, are exciting precisely because they take Alicia out of the family. There are no two places more different than the banquette in the restaurant and the matrimonial bed. At this moment, I have images from many of the Spanish and Portuguese movies I've seen of a room with a huge bed, complete with looming headboard, a crucifix on the wall, and women dressed in black. For a moment we enjoy naming some of movies with our favorite scenes of pleasure morgues.

There's a relief in the room, because for the first time both Roberto and Alicia feel that they're getting somewhere and that they're touching some of the roots of what has been so stultifying in the last 3 years. It is becoming clear why the circumstantial explanations always fell short.

Roberto wants to understand what Alicia means by "leaving home." Is it the domestic activities that Alicia needs to get away from? No. It is not the activities, it's the bed, and what one is *supposed* to do in that bed. In her mind, one is not allowed to experience pleasure in that bed. Women who experience pleasure are "*putas.*" Roberto grasps why she always comes on to him in outside places.

Now that we have understood that in order for Alicia to put the "X" back in "sex" she needs to leave the home, we explore together the many ways they can do so. Alicia has a fervent imagination. As Roberto says, "she's a creative act"; she refers to him as a "great audience." Her rich fantasy life has helped her circumvent the pitfalls of the prohibitions of her upbringing. Our fantasies combine the uniqueness of our personal history with the broad sweep of the collective imagination. Our flights of fancy bridge the gap between the possible and the permissible. Fantasy is the alchemy that turns this jumble of psychic ingredients into the gold of erotic arousal.

We explore erotic spaces they can introduce into their relationship, all the while living in their tiny studio. Remembering their 2-year long-distance relationship, I suggest they bring back some of the very modes of communication that were so electrifying back then. I suggest that they create separate e-mail addresses, ones that can not be used for domestic chores. This e-mail address exists outside of the family, so there is no need to navigate the two realms of experience: sex and family. It segregates the erotic into a sacred space, one exclusively reserved for erotic exchanges between them—their thoughts, memories, fantasies, and seductions. I point out that it is not meant to be a correspondence about the problems in their relationship, it is meant to be a space for play. I want them to use cyberspace to elicit curiosity, a sense of intrigue, and a kind of wholesome anxiety. Writing has many advantages over talking. You get to say your fill, craft your response, and give voice in writing to things your lips dare not utter. It provides a built-in distance, and I hope this will help them dismantle the inhibitions. There is a difference between sitting next to someone and saying, "Want to go to a movie" and texting them from the bathroom, "Do you want to go to a movie?" It can instantly lift one from the matter-of-fact to a subtle frisson. In the past 2 weeks this intervention has worked well, and they have used the technological built-in distance and anonymity to tease each other with unpredictability, playfulness, and mystery—all key erotic ingredients.

I also go back to one of their cherished activities when the Atlantic prevented them from touching each other: phone sex. They joke with me, saying that their home is too small to imagine the Atlantic. But once again, we agree that they will not get out of their quandary through reason and understanding, but by the force of their imaginations, which will take them away from *la cama matrimonial* (the matrimonial bed).

I offer a few more suggestions. They can read out loud to each other selected erotic writings, something they previously enjoyed doing together. Alicia can take Roberto to the video store and choose movies that show the kinds of seductive plots she enjoys. While these initiatives lighten up the conversation, and usher in a sense of humor, they don't spark any more interest. I ask both of them to list the things they enjoy doing—a comprehensive list of all that gives them pleasure, nothing to do with sex. Roberto realizes that he has truncated himself to such an extent that he feels uninteresting. I encourage him to reconnect with his friends, his local pub, his soccer team—in short Roberto needs to get Roberto back. That too will create some psychological space that should be propitious for desire to kick in.

Another suggestion adapted from Gina Ogden (2008), is offered to them. "Sit face to face and complete the statement: 'I turn myself off when.... ' Take turns and try to go back and forth for at least 10 or even 15 responses."

Alicia answers, "I turn myself off when I log on to Facebook before going to sleep ... I turn myself off when I don't have time for myself ... when I bring up our problems and frustrations when we finally have time to be alone for an evening ... when I don't feel good about my body ... "

Roberto answers, "When I think how long it's been since we've had sex ... when I think about how I'm losing my hair ... when I am resentful of Alicia ... when I feel pressure to perform and powerless to please her."

They are then instructed to complete another sentence: "I turn myself on when.... "

Alicia says, "I turn myself on when I don't feel pressure to have sex ... when I take care of my body and looks ... when I think of our early years ... when I think of the great sex I have had with you and with previous boyfriends ... when I give myself permission to leave the house chores for later ... when I watch something that makes me get hot ... when I am proud of myself."

Roberto says, "When I've just taken a shower ... when I cook great meals ... when we are apart for a while ... when I look at porn ... when I feel good about some accomplishments ... when I look at beautiful women ... when I fantasize about my past ... when we are having fun going to the movies and walking the streets ... when I feel good about my looks."

The lesson to be learned from this exercise is that *we* are the ones responsible for our erotic energy, our sexual interest or lack thereof. If we are open, then we are more likely to feel desirable and desirous. Each of us makes choices: how not to let ourselves be shut down, and how to keep ourselves sexually open and available. Moreover, all the ideas are yours.

Commentary

For Roberto and Alicia, therapy is in full swing. After four sessions, the undercurrents of the sexual stalemate have been brought to light. From here on, we follow a two-pronged approach that navigates between understanding, and doing. New awareness and creative resources will jolt couples out of a state of complacency and helplessness, but the challenge every therapist faces is to ensure the lasting shelf life of the changes. Therapy runs the risk of following the Weight

Watchers trajectory: you gain the weight back as soon as you are out of the program.

Many of the internal tensions that crackle in the sexuality of Alicia and Roberto are located in the reverberations of their childhoods and in the cultural transmissions they internalized. A multilayered understanding, the motivation to change, and a good fit between the partners are necessary to sustain change. But that too is not a guarantee. I will be meeting with each of them alone to further probe the nuances of their predicament, but also to map ways to amp up their erotic pulse. The rhythm of the therapy is like a metronome—the needle points back and forth between the individual and the couple. Each partner brings memories, apprehensions, expectations, and judgments to the relationship. They are personal at first, but they always become relational later.

The topics of the individual sessions may be the same; the conversations will not. For example, the issue of seduction is high on the list for both Alicia and Roberto. I will explore this with each partner and will translate for the other afterward. I think that for Alicia, like many women, seduction is key. It goes way beyond a simple string of compliments and flattery. Seduction acknowledges that there is no automatic yes, that sex is not a given, an a priori entitlement to the other. Seduction recognizes the other as a free agent who can respond overtly, or suggestively, or choose to ignore it altogether. What matters is that the receiver is free, not coerced in any way. This need for autonomy and freedom is essential to desire. For some women it is difficult to respond when their partner initiates. The dance I have seen goes as follows: He initiates, she pulls back, a while later (5 minutes, an hour, the next morning) she initiates, and then he welcomes her and their bodies swiftly interlace. Quite often, though, he responds to her approach by framing it as a power dynamic. He is hurt, interprets her advances as a power maneuver where sex can take place only on her terms, is angry that she will not take him in when he wants to, but only when it suits her.

To my mind, this is a misunderstanding of the conflict. For Alicia, and for many women, accepting his advances blurs the line between giving and giving in. The refusal, the partner's respect for that refusal, and then the free return are the tortuous way some women need to take to experience the autonomy of their desire. It is important to stress that the manouver is not about power over, but an attempt to delineate separateness, to ascertain ownership of desire. The lyrics of this song are as follows: "If I respond to you, I feel that I am giving in. How can I do what you want and feel that I want it too? The only way I know it is my free will is if I come toward you alone. If the coast is totally clear, all mine, then I know it is totally my desire. Otherwise, I can't hold on to my own wanting in the presence of a strong wanting on your part. When I initiate sex, I know I want it, when you initiate sex, I know you want it. I wish to find a way for my desires to live side by side with yours, not needing to ignore yours as a way to protect mine from the fear of obliteration."

Over the years I have come to recognize the value of this interpretation. If Roberto accepts it, he will be able to play, take risks, create anticipation, and know that Alicia's entanglements with her desire are not meant as a rejection of him. She needs to say "NO" so that she can then say "Yes," and this quest for free choice is not a statement about him. Helping Roberto out of the crucible of rejection and helping Alicia grasp the conflict of autonomy will be separate conversations at first. Then once these concepts have been assimilated they will be discussed together.

My teacher, Salvador Minuchin, once likened therapy to sculpting. I recall him saying that first you tackle the raw material, and you carve out gross shapes. These are dramatic moves, big chunks fall off, there is noise, instant change. But then comes the long, tedious period of chiselling, where you steadily go over and over the small gestures, trying to carve the lasting shape, the details, the enduring. That is the middle phase of therapy, the longest one, and there is hard work, but it isn't very dramatic. The commitment to the project, the ability to overcome frustrations, delighting in the glimpses of the envisioned possibilities are all part of the course. The finale, followed by the unveiling, is a rare bliss.

I would like for Roberto and Alicia to experience sex as pleasurable, inviting, and not dutiful. If we continue and chisel away, they stand a good chance to find a space where they can revere the erotic and delight in its irreverence. Nevertheless, I will tell them that all couples go through periods where desire is dormant, that erotic intensity waxes and wanes, and that desire can suffer periodic eclipses and intermittent disappearances. But given sufficient attention, they'll learn to bring it back. Eroticism in the home requires active engagement and willful intent. Committed sex is premeditated sex. It is an ongoing resistance to the message that marriage is serious, more work than play, that passion is for teenagers. We must unpack our ambivalence about pleasure and challenge our pervasive discomfort with sexuality, particularly in the context of family. Complaining of sexual boredom is easy and conventional. Nurturing eroticism in the home is an act of open defiance.

REFERENCES AND BIBLIOGRAPHY

Bader, M. J. (2002). *Arousal: The secret logic of sexual fantasies*. New York: St. Martin's.

Giddens, A. (1992). *The transformation of intimacy: Sexuality, love and eroticism in modern societies*. Stanford, CA: Stanford University Press.

Kipnis, L. (2003). *Against love: A polemic*. New York: Pantheon.

Mitchell, S. A. (2002). *Can love last?: The fate of romance over time*. New York: Norton.

Morin, J. (1995). *Erotic mind*. New York: HarperCollins.

O'Connor, D. (1986). *How to make love to the same person for the rest of your life and still love it*. London: Virgin.

Ogden, G. (2008). *The return of desire: A guide to recovering your sexual passion*. Boston: Trumpeter.

Perel, E. (2003, May/June). Erotic intelligence: Reconciling sensuality and domesticity. *Networker*.

Perel, E. (2006). *Mating in captivity: Reconciling The Erotic and the Domestic*. New York: HarperCollins.

Person, E. S. (1988). *Dreams of love and fateful encounters: The power of romantic passion*. New York: Norton

Schnarch, D. (1997). *Passionate marriage*. New York: Henry Holt.

Tiefer, L. (1995). *Sex is not a natural act and other essays*. Boulder, CO: Westview Press.

Chapter 3

Using Crucible Therapy to Treat Sexual Desire Disorders

David Schnarch

Over several decades of writing, teaching, and conducting therapy, David Schnarch has developed a unique approach to treating sex and relationship problems—an approach he terms Crucible therapy. While this approach fosters self-differentiation and self-regulation as well as the ability to live and love within a committed relationship, Schnarch's therapy is far-reaching in its use of confrontation, self-exploration, and personal challenge.

Schnarch believes that low and high desire are changeable positions within a relationship system and are not stable characteristics of a single individual. He notes that high- and low-desire partners are similar in differentiation, but the low-desire partner always controls sexual frequency and access. And while desire conflicts are inevitable and highly prevalent, they frequently lead to major rifts in relationships because "you can't agree to disagree with your partner about having sex."

In this chapter, he beautifully illustrates how he treats a couple in which the male partner avoids sexual intimacy. By using the "two-choice dilemma" (a situation where you want two choices but you get only one) as an organizing focus of treatment, Schnarch confronts the couple with their unspoken agendas and internal resistances to change. In this case, the husband embraces two contradictory wishes: "I don't want to have sex, but I want to be married to someone who wants sex" and "I agreed to monogamy, but now I want to change it to celibacy." The therapy centers on the resolution of these dilemmas.

David Schnarch, PhD, is Director of the Crucible Institute and the author of landmark books on sexual desire, including *Constructing the Sexual Crucible, Passionate Marriage, and Resurrecting Sex.* His latest book is *Intimacy & Desire.*

Modern treatment of sexual desire problems dates back to the 1970s with the work of Masters and Johnson, Helen Singer Kaplan, and others. Crucible® integrated sexual–marital therapy offers totally new ways to conceptualize and treat sexual desire problems. A crucible is a test of the most decisive kind, a challenge to your integrity and core values arising from powerful emotional and situational forces. A crucible is also a resilient container used in metallurgy to contain high-temperature chemical reactions. These definitions describe clients' personal experience and the level of intensity at which Crucible therapy operates.

Unlike other sex and marital therapy approaches, Crucible therapy is rooted in Bowenian differentiation theory (Bowen, 1978). Differentiation is the ability to balance attachment in relationships with self-direction and self-regulation, which boils down to "holding on to yourself" (keeping your emotional balance) in difficult interactions with others. Crucible therapy differs dramatically from Bowen therapy in its application of differentiation to intimacy and emotional relationships, its greater intensity, and its use of collaborative confrontation.

According to Crucible therapy, "marriage is a people-growing machine" driven by differentiation (Schnarch, 1991). The "gears" of the people-growing processes are described in a lexicon of coined terms: For example, poorly differentiated partners depend on a *reflected sense of self* (acceptance, validation, and empathy from others) and *anxiety regulation through accommodation* (regulating personal anxiety interpersonally through self-presentation and false agreement) from each other. They extract this through *other-validated intimacy* (partners are expected to accept and validate each other's disclosures). However, dependence on other-validated intimacy leads to *emotional gridlock* (impasse situations), which pushes partners to shift to *self-validated intimacy* (validating one's own disclosures without expecting acceptance from the partner) and become more differentiated through their struggles to do this (Schnarch, 1991, 1997,

2002, 2009). *Intimacy & Desire* details couples' inevitable struggles over intimacy, sex, and desire, and ties them to the processes of intrapersonal and interpersonal differentiation woven throughout monogamous love relationships.

Crucible therapy is also identifiable by what it does not do. It rejects (1) the diagnostic framework of "hypoactive" or "inhibited" sexual desire (ISD); (2) Kaplan's (1979) biological drive perspective and treatment approach; (3) the paradigm of "sex and desire are natural functions"; (4) "desire-phase disorders," a concept that emphasizes initiatory receptivity and assertiveness; and (5) the pathological view of people with low sexual desire enshrined in contemporary treatment and the DSM and ICDM diagnostic frameworks (Schnarch, 2000).

Instead, this therapy posits a completely different paradigm:

1. It approaches desire as a capacity that can be developed, rather than an inhibited drive.
2. It focuses on personal and relational growth (becoming more differentiated) rather than removing "blockages."
3. It focuses on desire for one's partner and desire *during* sex, rather than desire for sex, per se.

Most important for this chapter:

4. It approaches desire as a systemic relationship process, rather than a personal characteristic and individual diagnosis.
5. It steps outside the common linguistic and conceptual framework of "the identified patient and the asymptomatic partner."

CRUCIBLE PRINCIPLES ABOUT DESIRE PROBLEMS

Basic principles of Crucible therapy include the following:

• *Principle 1: One of the strongest determinants of human sexual desire (if not the strongest) is the process of developing and maintaining a phenomenological self.* At some point in human evolution, the human self emerged and sexual desire was irrevocably changed. About 1.6 million years ago, the struggles of emerging selfhood gradually began to outweigh biological imperatives, gene distribution strategies, or hormonal drives in determining sexual desire and sexual behavior.

- *Principle 2: Normal healthy people in good relationships have sexual desire problems.* *Intimacy & Desire* provides the first cohesive explanation for why, sooner or later, normal couples have sexual desire problems: it's due to the natural processes of differentiation. Couples arrive at this point from many different paths. When couples are emotionally gridlocked over intimacy (described above), desire fades. Principle 5 (below) states that normal interpersonal dynamics surrounding sexual desire create emotional gridlock and sexual desire problems, in and of themselves. Poorly differentiated couples develop emotional gridlock more quickly, more intensely, and more pervasively, and this holds true for sexual desire problems too. Being poorly differentiated is a nonpathological, normal state for individuals and couples.

- *Principle 3: "Low-desire partner" and "high-desire partner" are positions in a relationship system and are not reducible to individual characteristics (like biological drive, genetics, sexual preferences, family history, religious training, unconscious processes, or negative childhood experiences).* In contrast to earlier approaches to sexual desire problems, low-desire partners are not regarded as pathological, sexually inhibited, or emotionally blocked. They are not presumed to be more impaired or less differentiated than high-desire partners. People who have high libido and love sex are frequently shaped into occupying the "low-desire partner" position in their relationship by natural differentiation processes and/or their partner's behavior.

- *Principle 4: The low-desire partner and the high-desire partner do not differ in differentiation.* Crucible theory says people pick partners at the same level of differentiation. Moreover, because "low-desire partner" and "high-desire partner" are positions in a relationship, they do not differ in differentiation. Research indicates there is no reason to assume the low-desire partner's lower desire results from being less differentiated, sexually experienced, or interested, or likewise, more inhibited, emotionally damaged, or angry and withholding (Schnarch & Regas, 2008).

- *Principle 5: The low-desire partner always controls sex.* The high-desire partner makes the initiations, and the low-desire partner decides which ones to accept. This gives the low-desire partner de facto control of sex (excluding rape, emotional or physical battering, and places where women do not control their own bodies).

This approach views sexual desire problems as co-constructed interpersonal sociobiological and neurobiological events. They are driven by the way human differentiation and human sexuality are entwined today, and how they became entwined over the course of human evolution. The human brain and human sexual desire have co-developed for over a million years, shaping human nature and intimate relationships as our complex phenomenological "self" emerged. As a result, issues of adult "self" development (differentiation) greatly shape sexual desire in committed relationships, through developments like emotional gridlock and other relational processes. One reason normal healthy couples have sexual desire problems is because emotional gridlock dampens sexual desire, and emotional gridlock is virtually inevitable.

The politics of reflected sense of self steer the course of sexual desire in committed relationships (and extramarital affairs). In the early stages of relationships, desire is enhanced by partners supporting each other's reflected sense of self through other-validated intimacy. But sexual desire evaporates when couples battle out the predictable differentiation-driven self-development wars of *"Who do I belong to, me or you?!"* and *"I want to be with you, but don't tell me what to do!"* Power and control fights trump estrogen, testosterone, oxytocin, and libido every time. The same lack of differentiation (reflected sense of self) that spurs desire early in relationships also kills desire later on. The normal healthy battles of selfhood, which invariably occur in love relationships, make sexual desire problems a virtual certainty for normal healthy couples.

This view that sexual desire problems are normal is borne out by research conducted on the *DatelineNBC.com* website in 2006. When Dateline NBC devoted an hour of national prime-time coverage to couples undergoing Crucible therapy for sexual desire problems, over 27,500 people completed an online survey within 48 hours. *Sixty-eight percent reported sexual desire problems*: "Sex is dead" (13%); "Sex is comatose and in danger of dying (22%), or "Sex is asleep and needs a wake-up call" (33%). Only 22% reported, "Sex is alive and well," and just 10% said, "Sex is robust, erotic, and passionate."

PREVALENCE OF DESIRE PROBLEMS IN CLINICAL PRACTICE

More then half the cases I see involve couples who have sexual desire problems. Frequently this is not their presenting issue. Not because they are hiding or denying it. It's because they have other serious relationship difficulties: Many are on the verge of divorce; some are separated. Most have repeated disastrous arguments. Any prior collaborative alliance no longer exists. Sometimes sexual desire problems created this. Other times sexual desire was a casualty of emotional warfare.

Relationships frequently blow up over sexual desire problems. It's not just that sexual desire is so incredibly important to people, but that couples handle sexual desire problems so poorly. Likewise, conventional marital therapy wisdom fails when applied to sexual desire problems: You can't agree to disagree with your partner about having sex. And by the time you compromise and negotiate your way into bed, your desire is gone.

In half the heterosexual cases referred to me, the man is the low-desire partner. This may indicate men are as likely as women to be the low-desire partner in severe or difficult cases, since this constitutes the bulk of my practice. However, for clinical and theoretical reasons, I believe this is a more accurate picture of sexual desire problems in general.

CASE EXAMPLE: MR. AND MRS. DONNER

Initial Presentation

At the outset, both Mr. and Mrs. Donner said they were interested in treatment. Mr. Donner said he thought his desire was lower than that of most men, and he didn't want to lose his marriage. Mrs. Donner hoped treatment would improve their intimacy (in and out of bed) as well as their sexual frequency.

Mr. Donner (age 38) and Mrs. Donner (age 37) had been together for 15 years and married for 12. They had two children, ages 11 and 9. He was senior accountant in a large auditing firm. She resumed teaching high school when the children didn't need her as much as they had before.

Mr. Donner said he came from a home with an angry father. He thought this was why he was afraid of Mrs. Donner's temper. She exploded intermittently when they failed for months on end to have sex. Mrs. Donner said her father was often gone and her mother was an alcoholic. By her description, she was the classic "parentified child." She had several boyfriends in college and enjoyed sex with them. Mr. Donner rarely dated and had few sexual encounters.

When Mr. and Mrs. Donner first met, he was smitten with her.

Their sex was good and frequent. It tapered off when they moved in together, but they still had sex four or five times a month. This declined to once or twice a month by their third year together. Mrs. Donner attributed the decline to growing tension in their relationship at that time: They got married after Mrs. Donner presented Mr. Donner with the choice of getting married or breaking up because she wanted to have children. After their first child was born, sex declined further. But Mr. Donner seemed eager to have a second child, and Mrs. Donner agreed. After their second child was born, sex just about stopped.

Two years later, Mrs. Donner pushed to seek treatment but Mr. Donner refused. He did, however, agree to work on their problem. Several years later, the situation was unchanged. At that point, Mrs. Donner presented Mr. Donner with the choice of therapy or divorce.

Prior Treatment

Mr. and Mrs. Donner sought help from a local therapist who had a reputation for treating sexual problems. Mrs. Donner had read *Passionate Marriage* and wanted the kind of therapy described there. According to Mr. and Mrs. Donner, the therapist described her approach as "a combination of marital therapy, Masters and Johnson, and David Schnarch." Mr. and Mrs. Donner were prescribed communication skills, active listening activities, and nongenital and genital sensate focus exercises. "Dates" and text messaging were encouraged. Mrs. Donner was allowed to ask for sex, but Mr. Donner retained the right to refuse if he felt pressured.

Their therapist also directed Mr. and Mrs. Donner to open separate bank accounts, and develop separate friends, hobbies, and interests. With her encouragement, Mr. Donner attended a men's group for several months, and Mrs. Donner went on a weekend trip with her girlfriends. The therapist proposed that these pursuits would reduce the emotional fusion between them, and the "emotional vacation" from their daily interactions might stimulate Mr. Donner's desire. During this time they "dated" once a week, and in fact, sex improved. They had sex about once a week during 6 months of therapy. Mrs. Donner took this as a sign things were improving, and when Mr. Donner wanted to stop treatment she agreed.

Because the therapist talked about differentiation, couched interventions in the language of differentiation, and had Mr. Donner read *Passionate Marriage*, Mr. and Mrs. Donner thought she knew how to do differentiation-based therapy. But the hallmark of differentiation-based therapy is not discussions, readings, or insights about the process, it's *harnessing the differentiation process* by how therapy is conducted. In many successful cases, differentiation is never explicitly mentioned because the therapist's position in the therapeutic system drives the process, rather than the introduction of a concept. For instance, in Crucible therapy the therapist must maintain a well-differentiated stance. This is lost when "bans" (e.g., prohibiting intercourse) and prescriptions are given (e.g., separate bank accounts, sensate focus exercises, more sex), because these create unbalanced alliances with partners who have different motivations. Moreover, these activities are no longer self-defining acts ("differentiating moves") because clients are doing what they've been told to do.

When therapy ended, Mr. and Mrs. Donner's old patterns, sexual and otherwise, quickly reemerged because they had accomplished little in terms of differentiation. They went back to having sex once a month because this was all Mr. Donner wanted. Their arguments and problematic interactions returned, and Mr. and Mrs. Donner were demoralized.

It's not hard for treatment to produce *pseudo*differentiation and short-term increments in sexual frequency. Poorly differentiated people function better when they get a little emotional or physical distance *and/or* receive validation and positive reinforcement from their mate or therapist. Mr. and Mrs. Donner's prior therapy capitalized on this. But the hallmark of solid differentiation is its resilience across time and circumstance, especially when people and situations discourage the effort.

Mr. and Mrs. Donner returned to their therapist, who told them they were too emotionally fused for Mr. Donner to have desire. She proposed they extend their "emotional vacation" to living separately for a while. Mr. and Mrs. Donner refused and terminated with her shortly thereafter. They returned to their pattern of sex once every month or two. A year later they sought treatment with me because Mrs. Donner again presented the ultimatum of treatment or divorce.

Case Considerations: Treating Prior Treatment Failures

In my experience, sexual desire problems are no more difficult to treat than common sexual dysfunctions, which are not very difficult at all.

I attribute this to Crucible therapy's ability to handle (1) conflict, (2) failure, and (3) demoralization, which invariably surface with sexual problems. In conventional therapy, conflict interferes with couples agreeing to do sensate focus and active-listening exercises, and usually increases treatment failure.

I find couples' prior failures in treatment seriously complicate matters, especially when they believe they previously received adequate treatment from a qualified expert. My clients are sensitized to and demoralized by the conceptual, dynamic, and strategic pitfalls of conventional sexual desire treatment. The low-desire partner presumes he or she will be pressured to have more sex. The high-desire partner anticipates being pressured to accept less frequency or passion than he or she wants. Both partners expect one of two scenarios: I'll align with the high-desire partner and try to instill desire in the low-desire partner through prescribed activities. Or, I'll align with the low-desire partner and put a ban on sex, or put the low-desire partner in control of sexual initiations. In practice I do neither one, but couples wonder which of these unworkable strategies I'll employ, and whose interests I'll sell out.

Couples who previously failed in treatment are more doubtful about their choice of partner and the health of their relationship. They are more anxious in bed and in therapy, their emotions are labile, and they are depressed. They overreact and lock into (or avoid) arguments. They give up easily when things don't go smoothly.

Crucible therapy helps clients (1) maintain as more stable (solid) sense of self, (2) regulate their own anxiety and soothe their own heart, (3) remain nonreactive (but not indifferent) to their partner's anxiety and reactions, and (4) persevere through difficult times to accomplish their goals. It counteracts demoralization through interventions that rapidly accelerate treatment.

Treatment Course

Medical evaluation revealed no physiological, hormonal, or pharmacological cause for Mr. Donner's low sexual desire. Mr. and Mrs. Donner attended the Marriage & Family Health Center's Intensive Therapy Program located in Evergreen, Colorado, for three "intensives" 6 months apart, plus 3-hour telephone sessions every 3 to 4 weeks between intensives. Each intensive involved 16 to 20 hours of therapy over a 4-day period. Crucible therapy can be delivered in hourly weekly sessions, but the Intensive Therapy Program is especially designed for difficult couples who travel a long distance for treatment.

After their previous therapy ended, Mr. Donner took the position of "saying no to sex" in the name of becoming more differentiated. Mr. Donner thought I was going to support his position because he said this was his attempt to differentiate from his wife. Mrs. Donner said she wouldn't tolerate it anymore. Mr. Donner wanted me to extract a commitment from her to "work on their differentiation." I told him I was supporting his differentiation by *not doing* what he was asking.

Mr. Donner became upset and anxious, feeling that he was faced with a decisive choice about having sex. He framed his dilemma as *"Should I give in to save my marriage?"* I said this was not about giving in; it was about the best in him standing up to save his marriage. By going over the details of their early sexual relationship, I developed a revealing picture of both individuals and their relationship (an "elicitation window", Schnarch, 1991). It emerged that Mr. Donner "let" Mrs. Donner seduce him, thinking this would soon stop and their relationship would become platonic. He didn't inform her because, according to Mr. Donner, he was enjoying her affections at that point.

Accordingly, I organized part of Mr. and Mrs. Donner's therapy around the approach's material on *two-choice dilemmas* (wherein you want two choices, but you get only one). I told Mr. Donner he wasn't getting anywhere because he understated his situation. I described one of his two-choice dilemmas as *"I don't want to have sex, but I want to be married to someone who wants sex!"* Then I pointed out another one: *"I agreed to monogamy, but now I want to change it to celibacy!"*

Some clients who are avoiding their two-choice dilemmas like these "interpretations"—but continue to dodge. There's nothing magic about telling someone he has a two-choice dilemma. Instead I had to circumvent Mr. Donner's attempts to avoid confronting his situation. I also had to focus treatment on enhancing this couple's differentiation as individuals and as partners and reduce their emotional fusion. This, in turn, required constantly maintaining a balanced collaborative alliance with Mr. and Mrs. Donner. In part, I did this by making "isomorphic" interventions that simultaneously impacted *both* partners in ways helpful to each of them. I worked hard to develop a relationship with each of them as individuals, and our collaborative alliance helped them hear difficult things from me.

Crucible therapy calls this "working the lead," the skill and artistry of differentiation-based therapy. For instance, Mr. Donner said he needed more time to decide which way he wanted to resolve his two-choice dilemmas. I confronted him with the idea that he wanted more time to *not* decide. Mr. Donner said he had fears of abandonment from Mrs. Donner's threat to leave him. I told Mr. Donner he didn't form relationships; instead he took prisoners. He didn't like what I was saying, or what I was doing by saying it, but he didn't lose sight of the fact that I was trying to help him.

I told Mr. Donner he *"wanted to be wanted, but didn't want to want."* This is my way of stating a common two-choice dilemma in sexual desire problems (Schnarch, 1991). On the one hand, he wanted Mrs. Donner to desire and pursue him, because it made him feel desirable and valued when she did (reflected sense of self), and he became anxious when she lost interest (anxiety regulation through accommodation). On the other hand, Mr. Donner wouldn't tolerate the vulnerability of wanting Mrs. Donner more than she wanted him, even though he tried to keep her in this position for years. On top of this, not only did he lack desire, he wasn't interested in having more desire for these and other reasons.

All of this was wrapped up in my single statement, and it hit Mr. *and* Mrs. Donner like a ton of bricks, but in different ways. Mr. Donner was blasé talking about desire, but approaching desire as *wanting* changed the playing field. I pointed out that Mr. Donner got married—and had sex—because he didn't want to lose Mrs. Donner, not because he wanted her. His prior strategic straddle position, *"I want my wife, but I don't want sex,"* evaporated. The issue wasn't did he want sex, the issue was did he want *her?*

I also said his "not wanting to want" didn't start in this marriage. It was in place by the time he went to college. I left open where this might have come from, and noted aloud I knew nothing about his childhood or family. I knew I had struck a nerve, but Mr. Donner didn't pick up on this, and we stayed focused on his two-choice dilemmas.

My work with Mrs. Donner was equally intense and challenging, which counterbalanced my interventions with Mr. Donner, and maintained a balanced collaborative alliance that facilitated differentiation. I confronted Mrs. Donner about her emotional neediness and how she depended on getting a positive reflected sense of self from her husband. She was so desperate to be married, she had married a man who never chose her. She settled for being accepted and needed, but not wanted. Mr. Donner's misrepresentations that he wanted to have sexual desire had been enough to keep her in the marriage for years.

Mrs. Donner could see how she lied to herself and sold herself out. She knew it wasn't that he had no desire for sex. He had no desire for her. She hadn't wanted to admit it to herself, because then she'd have to deal with it. She also realized she had been "had." Mr. Donner frequently manipulated her through her need for validation.

When Mrs. Donner confronted herself, she told Mr. Donner she wouldn't settle for not being wanted. If he really didn't want her, then she wanted a divorce. This was not like her previous attempts to get him to validate her, or force him to have sex. This was not an infantile woman feeling hurt by not getting a positive reflected sense of self. Mrs. Donner was shifting from a reflected sense of self to a solid sense of self, triggered by acute and painful self-confrontation. Now she was willing to see the truth; she'd decide for herself whether he wanted her or not. At this point, Mr. and Mrs. Donner finally reached critical mass (Schnarch, 1991).

Treatment Outcome

Mr. Donner tried to keep his marriage going the way he wanted for as long as he could. Only when he realized he couldn't do this any longer did he begin to really deal with his situation. Mr. and Mrs. Donner both went through a "dark night of the soul." When Mr. Donner tried to slide by or sell out, I confronted him on it. Mrs. Donner didn't need much confrontation. This alone could have unbalanced my alliance with them. However, Mr. Donner took my moves as collaborative rather than adversarial because of our preceding therapy. The same interventions in a different (less-differentiated) therapy would have had different impacts.

I didn't permit a "just do it" approach. That would have allowed Mr. Donner to avoid his *not wanting to want*, and interfered with Mrs. Donner validating herself enough to think she was worth wanting. Instead I helped them both go through their crucible and face their two-choice dilemmas.

Mr. Donner finally confronted himself about never choosing Mrs. Donner. He had been too insecure to choose. He feared the control she would have in his life, and he couldn't handle the vulnerability, tension, and self-denial involved in loving someone. He accepted the idea this came from his growing up, but our focus stayed on the present situation and necessary decisions, rather than talking about his feelings and disappointments with his parents. This maintained their crucible and kept the differentiation process alive. When we reprocessed Mr. Donner's childhood later in therapy, his account of his life story changed.

Mr. Donner "took the hit" and acknowledged he had never chosen Mrs. Donner. He also said he didn't find her sexually attractive anymore. He acknowledged not respecting her because she sold herself out to get people—him, her mother, and friends—to like her. Rather than getting "wounded," Mrs. Donner stepped up and acknowledged this was true. Their unsettling interchanges in uncharted territory created the most intense intimacy Mr. and Mrs. Donner ever experienced. The more Mr. Donner experienced his wife as a separate person who could hold on to herself with him, the more he found her sexually interesting. Their growing self-respect and respect for each other led to new sexual initiations and longer foreplay, which grew out of the more solid self and greater self-regulation they developed through the therapy.

When Mr. Donner started initiating, Mrs. Donner was hypervigilant to detect if he was trying to buy her off or contain the situation. But their relaxed emotional connection from doing *hugging till relaxed* and *heads on pillows* began to deepen (Schnarch, 1991, 1997, 2002, 2009). *Hugging till relaxed* is a multipurpose long-duration hug focused on enhancing differentiation and intimacy, rather than making one's partner feel soothed and secure. It involves standing on your own two feet and soothing yourself down while being physically and emotionally engaged with your partner. *Heads on pillows* uses nonsexual long-duration eye gazing to accomplish similar goals, in an "in bed" context couples associate with sex, anxiety, and conflict. Although I am known for creating both tools, I didn't lose my well-differentiated stance by prescribing them. Mr. Donner and Mrs. Donner read about them in *Passionate Marriage,* and when Mr. Donner asked if I thought he should do them, I told him to make up his own mind. I framed this as his needing to decide who he wanted to be and become it—and he wasn't going to do that by following my instructions.

When Mr. Donner suggested doing *heads on pillows* several days later, he and Mrs. Donner knew this was on his own initiative. Looking into his eyes, she could see more openness and availability. Their sex became more meaningful, more relaxing, and less anxious. They got along better and they looked better. Mr. and Mrs. Donner showed more sexual desire before and during sex. Their individual functioning improved, as did their sexual frequency and relationship satisfaction. Intimacy increased in and out of bed.

I remained cautious about Mr. Donner's progress until it became clear he was involved and benefiting from therapy. The couple engaged in *hugging till relaxed* and *heads on pillows* for increasing periods, eventually settling into a pattern of 20 minutes three or four times a week. They reported deep relaxation in an intimate context. They learned to regulate their emotions and keep their reactivity under control when things didn't go well. They developed greater ability to function autonomously *and* be closer together, physically and emotionally.

Mr. and Mrs. Donner increased their differentiation and reduced their emotional fusion. In the process, they simultaneously activated multiple levels of brain function (e.g., sensory, motor, emotions, cognitions) in a densely layered, powerfully positive, high-meaning framework that involved their minds, bodies, and relationship with each other. These qualities of interaction are thought to contribute to brain plasticity and interpersonal neurobiological reorganization (Cozolino, 2002).

I knew they were progressing when I saw evidence of *brightening,* a softening of facial features and an appearance of aliveness, vitality, energy, and healthy countenance. Women look like they've had a face lift, and men look softer and more handsome. It's no mystery why couples resume having sex: they feel and look more attractive, and they are more attracted to each other. People who display brightening find their own eyes look clearer and brighter, their mental acuity is sharper, and their general and emotional intelligence increases. *Brightening* is identifiable by untrained observers. Other people find them more attractive and approachable too.

It is my belief that *brightening* reflects shifts in brain function. It happens too quickly and too pervasively to be simply learning. Couples who show brightening think differently and handle their emotions better. Their marriages become more stable and less anxiety driven. Partners become more relaxed, more considerate, and more direct with each other. Relationships with children, parents, or friends become richer, deeper, and more resilient. Parents report positive changes in their children. Clients' changes are relatively resilient under stress, as one might expect if their brains are functioning differently.

COMMENTARY

Emotionally fused couples have to reach critical mass to take significant steps in personal development. That's the level of anxiety and pressure necessary to create fundamental change in people and systems (e.g., marriage, families, organizations). The lower one's differentiation, the greater the anxiety and pressure required to reach critical mass. Intense levels of emotion, anxiety, and conflict are not a problem for Crucible therapy. Holding on to yourself in the midst of this *is* the therapy. Conflict in love relationships is how human beings naturally grow. Therapies that don't handle conflict well are therapies at odds with the way relationships operate.

The therapist's personal differentiation sets the upper limit of his or her effectiveness in treating sexual desire problems (or any psychotherapy, whether differentiation based or not): Couples whose level of anxiety and pressure required to reach critical mass exceeds their therapist's level of differentiation cannot significantly reduce their emotional fusion with that therapist.

Differentiation-based therapy is not as simple as applying the concept of differentiation. Raising people's differentiation doesn't occur by giving interpretations or prescribing situational changes. It is an arduous and intense process. Therapists' practical ability to facilitate clients' differentiation requires theoretical and clinical accuracy, as well as the ability to operate under pressure.

Bowen himself doubted people could raise their differentiation, especially without extreme effort. He didn't think bibliotherapy, communication, and empathy skills training or psychodynamic, insight-oriented, or emotion-based cathartic psychotherapy could do it. From years of doing "extreme effort" therapy, I am more optimistic than Bowen.

The impact of an intervention is co-created by clients and therapists. Much of that stems from the therapist's differentiation and his or her position in the interpersonal dynamics of treatment at that moment. Simply copying interventions described here will not produce differentiation-enhancing therapy. That's because (1) the client often gets around the therapist, (2) the therapist can't steer the intervention and keep it on track, (3) the therapist leads the client too much when making the move ("snare-trap therapy"), or (4) the therapist loses a differentiated clinical stance. My interventions came out of caring enough to confront people with their lives, rather than combatively trying to "beat clients at their own game" or "get them."

Moreover, their impact was greatly determined by the meaning frame and momentum I co-developed with these clients in preceding interactions.

Discussing differentiation and helping clients become more differentiated are two different things. The latter requires working the differentiation process in real time. Crucible therapy harnesses this process, sometimes without ever naming it explicitly.

Effectively treating sexual desire problems involves more than making the problems go away. It involves resolving them in ways that enhance both partners' personal development. I've come to believe this is why Nature ordained that the low-desire partner always controls sex and normal couples shall have sexual desire problems. Good treatment approaches this inevitable development in ways that fulfill its "purpose." This requires believing that marriage is a people-growing machine.

Working with differentiation doesn't complicate treatment, but makes it easier and more effective. It's much easier to resolve sexual desire problems when treatment lines up with how differentiation permeates sexual desire, sex, and intimacy in emotionally committed relationships. Sexual desire, differentiation, and our mind and brain are inextricably linked. Perhaps the question is no longer *"Can sexual desire problems be treated effectively?"* It is how effectively can sexual desire treatment create pervasive nonsexual changes?

REFERENCES

Bowen, M. (1978). *Family therapy in clinical practice.* New York: Jason Aronson.

Cozolino, L. (2002). *The neuroscience of psychotherapy: Building and rebuilding the human brain.* New York: Norton.

Kaplan, H. S. (1979). *Disorders of sexual desire and other new concepts and techniques in sex therapy.* New York: Brunner/Mazel.

Schnarch, D. M. (1991). *Constructing the sexual crucible: An integration of sexual and marital therapy.* New York: Norton.

Schnarch, D. M. (1997). *Passionate marriage: Sex, love, & intimacy in emotionally committed relationships.* New York: Norton.

Schnarch, D. M. (2000). Sexual desire: A systemic perspective. In S. R. Leiblum & R. C. Rosen (Eds.), *Principles and practices of sex therapy* (3rd ed.). New York: Guilford Press.

Schnarch, D. M. (2002). *Resurrecting sex: Resolving sexual problems and rejuvenating your relationship.* New York: HarperCollins.

Schnarch, D. M. (2009). *Intimacy & desire: Awaken the passion in your relationship*. New York: Beaufort Books.

Schnarch, D. M., & Regas, S. (2008). *Relationship between sexual satisfaction, sexual functioning and level of differentiation*. Paper presented at the annual conference of the American Association for Marriage and Family Therapy, Memphis, TN.

Chapter 4

The Canary in the Coal Mine

*Reviving Sexual Desire
in Long-Term Relationships*

Kathryn Hall

Kathryn Hall aptly observes that desire is the wish for something that one doesn't have. This may explain why sexual passion burns more brightly in forbidden relationships or those marked by obstacle or objection. Obligatory sex stifles desire.

In the case that follows, the client's explanation for her lack of desire is ascribed to her incestuous experiences as a child. It is true that sexual abuse is often a factor in complaints regarding sexual apathy or aversion. But equally significant are the erroneous beliefs regarding sexual desire and the client's internal voice forbidding her to decline sex for fear of losing her relationship. By receiving permission to say no to obligatory sex, Andrea is able to attend to, and be curious about, her own nascent sexual feelings. Therapy is not focused on increasing desire but rather on helping Andrea understand and appreciate her unique sexuality.

Unlike many of the cases described in this book, individual rather than couple therapy is provided. Individual therapy is sometimes quite effective, especially where there are long-standing issues that have not been resolved, such as a past history of sexual abuse or domestic violence.

Hall's major take-home message is that the therapist must not want the client to have sex more often than the client herself wants it. To impose an expectation that more frequent sex is the desirable outcome in cases involving sexual apathy is simply to reinforce an unacceptable standard.

Kathryn Hall, PhD, is in private practice in Princeton, New Jersey, and the author of a popular book on sexuality entitled *Reclaiming Your Sexual Self: How You Can Bring Desire Back into Your Life.*

"I wish I wanted to have sex, but I just don't." Problems with sexual desire are the most frequent complaint of women coming to my sex therapy practice, and yet sexual desire itself is probably the most misunderstood facet of sexual responding. Most women (and most of my clients complaining of sexual desire problems are women) believe that the problem resides within them. They believe that there is something wrong with them if they do not regularly experience spontaneous sexual desire for their partner, otherwise known as lust or feeling "horny." Most women report that they did at one time experience such feelings. The fact that they now do not is often troubling and distressing not only to them, but also to their partners: "I want to feel wanted too—I want to know that she desires me" is a frequent grievance. Because my clinical experience tells me that loss of sexual desire is different for men and women in both etiology and treatment, this chapter will be directed at sexual desire problems in women.

A common misconception is that men and women's sexuality is essentially the same, which leads to the belief that the experience of sexual desire should also be identical across gender. While the majority of men experience spontaneous sexual desire and think about sex a lot, most women do not, especially as they age and once they are in a long-term relationship. This change should not be diagnosed as a sexual dysfunction, although the couple's distress and difficulty adjusting to the change may be a focus of treatment. Loss of desire in romantic relationships is very stressful for Western couples, who tend to equate love with sexual desire. Couples in other cultures that distinguish between lust and love and do not rely on the former for initiating sexual activity do not frequently complain of low desire.

A linear model of sexual responding, wherein sexual desire is a necessary first step preceding sexual activity, does not reflect the reality of most women's experience. A pattern of responding that I have called the desire–arousal feedback loop (Hall, 2004) and Rosemary Basson (2007) has more eloquently described in her circular model of the sexual response cycle reflects the fact that sexual desire in women is often responsive rather than spontaneous. Sexual desire is not experienced only prior to sex, rather it is the wish, the motivation, and the physical urge to engage in sex (or more sex) that is often sparked by sexual arousal and that hopefully continues throughout a sexual encounter. Many women erroneously believe that they have a sexual desire disorder because they do not feel physically turned on prior to sex. Many women do report that they experience desire for sex once they are having sex. In other words, once they are aroused, often by direct touch, they want more sexual stimulation and when sex is over, they often wonder why they don't have sex more often. In these cases, one of the goals of treatment is to help women identify what could prompt their interest in having sex prior to arousal.

Desire is the wish for something that one doesn't have. This is why sexual desire remains high in relationships in which sex is either forbidden (premarital or extramarital relationships) or optional (dating, casual relationships) or where there is an obstacle such as distance, differing religious faiths, or familial objections. When sex is expected it often feels obligatory and then one can lose sight of desire, of wanting. It is difficult to experience want for something you already have, or indeed, must have. This is why sexual desire becomes problematic in many marriages and committed relationships.

Sexual desire is often like the proverbial canary in the coal mine, with the loss of desire being an early indication of trouble in a relationship. Because sexual desire is about connection, of all the sexual responses it will be especially sensitive to a disconnection in the couple bond. Sometimes, the loss of sexual passion is recognized as an indication of problems in the relationship. However, the usual course of desire disorders follows roughly the same story line: The person who first experiences the drop in sexual interest denies to herself that it is a problem. Once she can no longer deny it, she tries to deal with it on her own. She may try to hide it from her partner, often relying on a calendar for initiating or responding to sex. This calendar is based on avoiding her partner's anger rather than on sexual interest or desire: "If we don't have sex for a week, 2 weeks, 3 days ... my partner will be angry." The reason for the drop in desire is either unknown to the woman or is one that she will have trouble resolving on her own or with her partner. For example, while she may be aware that her lack of desire has to do with her feelings about the status of her relationship or her feelings about her partner, she may be unable or unwilling to discuss this with him or her. On the other hand, she may believe that her lack of desire has something to do with her own personal issues. She may believe that she is out of love with her partner, that she has intimacy problems, or that she has issues with sex. These self-statements are more likely if she has experienced a loss of desire in other relationships in the past. Once the lack of desire has become apparent in the relationship, it has likely been occurring for some time. Attempts to rectify the problem may result in additional disruption for the couple. It is not uncommon for a low-desiring woman to engage in sex solely to please or pacify her partner and therefore rush through sex and/or focus on her partner's pleasure at the expense of her own. This pattern will reinforce her belief that she does not desire and even really enjoy sex. When all else fails, a therapist may be consulted. As therapists, we are lucky when men or women or couples consult us at the first sign of trouble. But more often than not, we are the last resort.

Women with low sexual desire often hope that the problem may be hormonal. While many women reject this notion, they nonetheless feel a tremendous societal as well as interpersonal pressure to feel something (lust) that may not be realistic. So while they may not believe that the problem is hormonally based, they may want the solution to be. As an explanation a hormone imbalance alleviates the shame low-desiring women feel and reduces blaming within the relationship. The promise of a quick fix that does not require change in oneself or the relationship is almost irresistible. But this is why hormonal treatment will ultimately fail as a panacea for low sexual desire. While an initial rise in sexual activity often occurs with hormone therapy, much of this activity can be attributed to an improvement in the relationship and in one's outlook because of the attention being paid to the problem. Hence the large placebo effect evident in drug trials for sexual disorders (Bradford & Meston, 2007). Increased sexual activity may also occur in the beginning stages of sex therapy. Most often, however, clients wait anxiously to hear what is wrong with them or with their relationship. This negative anticipation precludes increased sexual interest and activity.

In heterosexual relationships it is usually the woman who loses sexual desire. It is often assumed that men's sexual desire, fueled by higher levels of testosterone, is stronger and therefore more resilient to a downturn in the emotional tone of the relationship. Men also tend to view sex as a way to reconnect with their partners; they see it as a route to intimacy, whereas women tend to view sex as an outcome of emotional closeness—or at least this seems to hold true in the majority of long-term relationships. The situation is more complicated in same-sex relationships. Why one member of a couple manifests the couple's distress through a lack of desire is often unclear. While this may simply be related to differences in innate levels of sexual drive that the individuals have, the loss of desire in one partner, and the couple's reaction to that loss, may shed real light on the inner workings of the relationship, in a way that it does not in heterosexual relationships. The couple that I have chosen to discuss will be instructive for both heterosexual and lesbian relationships.

Individuals and couples with low sexual desire are among the most challenging of our cases. Other sexual problems involve improving, changing, or enhancing sexual responses to sexual stimulation— not so in situations involving low desire. In these cases, individuals or couples expect to feel something in the absence of any direct or physical stimulation. Managing unrealistic expectations and dealing with the often acute shame one experiences for not being sexual are hurdles to treatment progress.

CASE EXAMPLE: ANDREA AND CRICKET

The first thing I noticed about Andrea was her beauty, and I initially thought it likely that she was more accustomed to being an object rather than an agent of desire. At age 46, she was tall, slim, and graceful. Her face was youthful and she had large blue eyes that gave her the look of a deer in the headlights. Her style of dress was best described as understated and she wore little makeup or jewelry. By the end of our first session it was obvious to me that Andrea had no awareness of herself as beautiful or sexual.

Andrea came to see me at the urging of her partner, Christine. Christine, affectionately called Cricket, was unhappy about the lack of sex in the relationship. Cricket and Andrea had been living together for about 7 years, but sex had been infrequent after the first year and had further diminished in frequency over the last 2 years. Andrea and Cricket had sex approximately once every 6 to 8 weeks. A huge fight and the threat of breaking up prompted Andrea to make an appointment for therapy. It is important to note that Andrea was not unhappy about the lack of sex but she was unhappy about the status of the relationship. "If I never had sex again, it would be okay with me. I just don't want to keep fighting about it. I know Cricket is right. I know that sex is an important part of a relationship, and I wish I felt that way about her. She deserves it, she really does."

Andrea and Cricket often fought about the lack of sex but now the arguing was becoming more frequent and more intense and

Cricket was threatening to end the relationship. Cricket, a psychotherapist herself, always wanted to "talk about the relationship." But to Andrea, the talking was tantamount to a recitation of the things that were wrong with her and she was tired of hearing about them. The reasons—or in Cricket's opinion, the excuses—regarding the lack of sexual activity were getting old. They were no longer working to assuage Cricket's hurt feelings or to convince her that Andrea truly loved her. Cricket had asked Andrea many times to go to therapy with her, but Andrea always refused. She did not want to feel "ganged up on by two therapists." Andrea finally called for an appointment with me after Cricket spent the preceding two nights on the living room couch.

The story Andrea told about her lack of desire could be summarized as follows: It is my own problem; it has nothing to do with my partner. I don't want to have sex now because I was sexually abused as a child.

Although infrequent, the sex that Andrea and Cricket had was routine and predictable. The two mutually agreed that sex could never occur before a workday and it could not happen late at night and it had to start and end in the bedroom. So sex was relegated to Saturday mornings. Cricket always initiated sex and insisted that she pleasure Andrea first. Routinely, sex ended when Andrea experienced an orgasm. When Andrea would attempt to reciprocate, Cricket would frequently assure her that it was "okay." This furthered Andrea's feeling that she was beholden to Cricket, in other words, the sexual experience increased her feeling of obligation rather than lessening it.

In terms of the sexual abuse, Andrea stated the following facts: She was abused when she was between the ages of 9 and 11 years by her father. Andrea's parents slept in separate rooms; her mother slept on the main floor as she had lupus and found climbing stairs tiring, and her father slept in the master bedroom next to Andrea's room. On many occasions Andrea went to snuggle in bed with her father, whom she identified as the more emotionally available parent. The first memory she had of the abuse was when she was about 9 years old and in bed with her father. He stroked her genitals under her nightgown and the touch felt good to Andrea—until she came to understand what it meant. Andrea reported that she then felt very guilty that she never did anything to stop it. "The truth is I didn't want him to stop. It felt good." The abuse ended when Andrea no longer went to sleep in her father's room; nonetheless, the guilt that she felt for her "participation" was very strong.

Unaware of her sexual orientation or indeed any sexual feelings, Andrea dated several boys in high school. She found it easy to resist the sexual advances of her boyfriends and she prided herself on being a "good girl." In college, however, she found the rules for being a "good girl" changed. Her virginity was now seen as a liability and she was eager to "get rid of it." She had several boyfriends in college but never really enjoyed sex. It wasn't until she was a junior that she had an inkling she was sexually attracted to women. After a few furtive and alcohol-aided sexual encounters with "a friend," Andrea realized that she was a lesbian.

Andrea's loss of desire was a pattern in her lesbian relationships. While she had no desire for sex in her past heterosexual relationships, the beginnings of her relationships with women were characterized by strong sexual interest and frequent sexual activity. Initially, Andrea experienced sex as pleasurable and engaged in a variety of activities including caressing, oral sex, and vaginal penetration with fingers, dildos, and vibrators. As her desire waned, Andrea would begin to restrict sexual activity, preferring a "let's just get it over with" attitude to a pleasure-oriented approach. Over time sex would become less varied, more infrequent, and less fun. As her desire for sex with her partner waned, Andrea would take on more of the household responsibilities and often found herself doing the majority of the cooking, cleaning, and home maintenance. During the evaluation she recognized that she was trying to "prove my worth or maybe express my love and interest" through avenues other than sex. Andrea believed that her lack of sexual interest was responsible for the breakup of her previous relationships.

Andrea was in a 10-year relationship that ended just before she met Cricket. This relationship was sexless for the last 4 years, which Andrea believed was by mutual consent. When her partner told her that she had been having an affair during that time, Andrea was devastated. Andrea met Cricket shortly thereafter and was charmed by her easygoing manner (as evidenced by her nickname) and they soon moved in together.

Andrea was not attracted to other women; she masturbated infrequently and felt guilty about it when she did, as if she were cheating her partner of her sexual energy. Because this same pattern of losing desire had happened in previous relationships at much younger ages, it did not appear to be a physical issue. As a health-conscious individual, Andrea had regular physical exams, Pap smears, and mammograms.

Treatment lasted almost 1 full year. Andrea was seen for 24 sessions on a weekly basis, then 2 sessions on a monthly basis and a follow-up session 3 months later. This last session was about 1 year after the initial evaluation.

The outcome of this case was very successful. Andrea experienced sexual desire for her partner; the relationship between the two women improved and Andrea felt increased self-esteem and overall satisfaction with her life. Cases of low sexual desire are not always resolved so well or so quickly (although many would not consider a year of therapy quick). Often the relationship improves and there is greater acceptance of the lack of desire. This case is instructive for what went well.

Case Formulation

Andrea was disconnected from her sexual desire and it was a problem for her in terms of maintaining intimate relationships. She viewed sex as something she needed to do to be in a relationship, to make her partner happy. It was not something she did for the pleasure of it. Given this, it was understandable that Andrea often acted as though she could trade off one duty for another—she could make up for the lack of sex by doing an extra few loads of laundry or mopping the kitchen floor. Andrea's lack of sexual desire for Cricket was likely facilitated by the following several factors:

1. *The guilt that she felt regarding the incest.* Andrea's understanding of the sexual abuse was that it was her fault—after all she had been the one to go into her father's bed, she had enjoyed the touching, and when she no longer sought her father out at night, the abuse stopped. It was easy for her as a child to assume that the sexual abuse was in her control and something that happened because she wanted it to. It is likely that Andrea suppressed her sexual feelings as an adolescent and as an adult because of the guilt associated with being a sexual agent.

2. *Sociocultural pressures to conform to a model of the "good girl."* While many women of Andrea's generation were subjected to the same societal pressures to regulate the sexual activities they engaged in with boys, Andrea may have been especially vulnerable to this pressure given her history of abuse, as well as having an ill mother and an emotionally needy father (which heightened her sense of responsibility). The fact that Andrea was unaware of her sexual

orientation meant that she had no sexually arousing experiences in adolescence, which further reduced her awareness of sexual arousal and desire.

3. *Relationship dynamics.* Although we know about the relationship only from Andrea's perspective, this does give us an important glimpse into the way that she experiences the relationship. From Andrea's description, it seemed that Cricket did not want sex for the sheer pleasure of it. Andrea was unable to give any indication of what Cricket's sexual interests were, apart from wanting to please Andrea. It was my working hypothesis that, as with many partners of low-desiring women, Cricket wanted to be wanted, but like many women, she was settling for being needed. However, Cricket was unwittingly playing into a dynamic that was inherent in Andrea's incest—an emotionally or sexually needy person being gratified by Andrea's sexual arousal and orgasm. In addition to a replay of the incest dynamic, the sexual experiences of Andrea and Cricket only served to increase Andrea's sense of obligation regarding sex—and the experience of sexual obligation is most often the death of desire.

Evaluation and Treatment

Treatment of sexual problems actually begins during the evaluation. In addition to a thorough assessment of the sexual complaint (including an individual sexual history and an examination of the couple dynamic) this is a good time for sex education. Explaining that women's sexual desire is often responsive rather than spontaneous alleviates the shame and blame that are often part of the presenting complaint. In Andrea's case, she clearly blamed herself for the sexual problems in the relationship. She attributed her low desire to her history of incest but this just made her feel damaged and helpless to change the situation. An important point in therapy happened during the initial evaluation when Andrea realized that she did experience sexual desire during sex. My questions regarding Cricket and why she did not want to receive sexual pleasure from Andrea allowed Andrea to question her original assumption that she was the only one in the couple with sexual issues.

Some of the critical issues that were addressed in therapy are discussed below. It is important to note that once raised, these issues were often discussed many times during the course of therapy. Andrea was seen individually, as this was her strong preference. I did not press to see Cricket even once during the evaluation because Andrea was very sensitive to feeling that Cricket knew how to be in a relationship and she did not. In other words, Andrea needed the time and space in therapy to discover her own feelings and desires (sexual and otherwise) regarding her self in relationship. Given that Cricket was a psychotherapist, the risk of Andrea feeling judged by two professionals was high. It is also my belief that one can work systemically with only one member of a couple. If one person changes, the nature of the dyad must necessarily change as a result. As therapy progressed and progressed well there was never a pressing need to invite Cricket in to therapy, nor did Cricket ever make her participation an issue.

Early on in therapy I shared with Andrea my clinical impressions from our initial sessions. I told Andrea that her lack of sexual desire appeared to be a reasonable response to her situation. Her relationship with Cricket was following a similar pattern of duty and obligation to that which began in her family of origin and continued in her subsequent romantic relationships. Duty and obligation understandably conflicted with her ability to experience desire. Reframing her lack of desire as an understandable response was a pivotal moment in therapy. It was not as she feared, that either there was something wrong with her, or worse, that she did not love Cricket. Understanding her lack of desire did not bring Andrea's desire back. What the reframing did was to eliminate Andrea's defensiveness and redirect the process of therapy with an eager and willing participant. Andrea came to therapy out of fear of losing her relationship with Cricket. She continued to come to therapy for her own growth.

In the initial evaluation, Andrea disclosed the sexual abuse, going into specific details when guided by my questions. It was essential for Andrea to disclose details to assure herself that I understood all that had occurred when we discussed the impact of the sexual abuse on her present sexuality. Helping Andrea comprehend how the abuse, and her understandable reaction to it, worked with other factors in her life to contribute to her current desire problems was a crucial part of therapy. This allowed Andrea to move from a position of helplessness and hopelessness—"I am damaged and there is nothing I can do about it"—to feeling hopeful and energized: "I learned about unhealthy sexuality, now I can learn and experience healthy adult sexuality. I can learn about my own sexual feelings and I can trust and enjoy them."

In the subsequent 2 weeks Andrea and Cricket had frequent (twice weekly) sex, without any increase in Andrea's desire or motivation other than to prove to Cricket that she was working in therapy.

I continued to affirm Andrea's right to say no to sex and we continued to explore her lack of desire in the context of the issues raised in the evaluation. It should be noted that when couples rush quickly back into having sex without making real changes in the relationship, they are often just engaging in another variation of obligatory sex (we are in therapy and so we should be doing something about sex). Indeed, the brief increase in sexual activity did not last.

As I continued to align with Andrea's right and inclination to say no to sex, I gave her the freedom to explore and discover her right and inclination to say yes. After several months of therapy, Andrea no longer felt defensive or hopeless and she was in a good position to explore her nascent interest in and/or motivation for sex. The fact that Andrea did feel desire during sex was a baseline as I encouraged Andrea to be curious about what else might elicit sexual interest, arousal, or desire. Curiosity reverses the avoidance of all things sexual that usually occurs in women with low desire. I utilized some of the techniques that are outlined in the book *Reclaiming Your Sexual Self* (Hall, 2004). The movie critique technique was one that worked well with Andrea, as she was an avid moviegoer. In this exercise, Andrea thought about several romantic films that she really liked and answered questions about them, including ones that instructed her to explore what it was about the relationship between the lovers that she found compelling as well as what happened during any sex scene that she found erotic. It did not matter to Andrea that most if not all of the movies involved heterosexual relationships; she still felt an interest in the key dynamics of the major players. In particular, she loved the old movies involving Spencer Tracy and Katharine Hepburn and she found their verbal sparring exciting, especially the fact that they didn't always have to give in and see each other's viewpoint. She was also drawn to the smart and sexy characters in the television series *The L Word*. In addition to personality factors, she noticed the women's bodies and their lingerie, their casual attitude toward sex, and the element of play that was often apparent. I was careful not to encourage or suggest to Andrea that she "try this at home." Therapy was an opportunity for Andrea to be curious without being committed to action. She did ask for suggestions on books and websites and I recommended two websites (*www.goodvibes.com* and *www.babeland.com*) as well as the book *The Guide to Getting It On* (Joannides, 2008). After reading through parts of the book, Andrea masturbated for the first time in many years, a practice she continued throughout therapy. Andrea reported feeling sexy but realized that in her relationship with Cricket she was not acting like a smart, sexy woman who was an equal with her partner. In therapy, Andrea and I role-played several interactions she had had in the past, or anticipated having in the future, with Cricket. Andrea practiced relating to her lover in a more confident and assertive way. Soon when Cricket wanted to talk, Andrea was either able to participate in a discussion representing her own point of view or she was able to say she did not want to talk at the moment. Andrea was also able to leave a conversation "agreeing to disagree." While she experimented and had support in therapy for making changes in the way she related to Cricket, she also became curious and began to experiment in the way she related sexually to Cricket. Andrea initiated sex on a few occasions, and during sex she began to be more assertive about what she wanted (and often this involved pleasuring Cricket). We also talked about slowing down the pace of sexual activity so that Andrea could attend to sexual feelings and desires as they arose during sex. We discussed both the concept and the techniques involved in building desire rather than sating sexual arousal with a quick orgasm.

When Andrea began to initiate sex, she found that contrary to her expectations, Cricket was not always ready or willing to have sex with her. This was a relief to Andrea and was instructive as well. Now that Andrea was sharing the initiation of sex, Cricket began to share the limit setting. Contrary to Andrea's fears, Cricket did not always want to have sex. At this point, I did some coaching with Andrea so she could begin to decipher and then to ask and check out her assumptions about what made Cricket want to have sex with her. Andrea realized that various emotional factors were responsible for Cricket wanting sex. Some of these emotions similarly motivated Andrea to seek out sex, among them a desire for intimacy, reconnecting after an absence or an argument, wanting to express love or to relax and be playful. Lust or spontaneous sexual desire was a rare occurrence for both Cricket and Andrea, a fact that was both new and reassuring to Andrea.

Toward the end of therapy, Andrea reported that other people had begun to take notice of her and she found herself the object of sexual attention from both men and women. Men (assuming she was single) asked her out and other lesbians flirted with her. This was a strong sign that Andrea had begun to integrate her sexuality into her life and personality in a meaningful and lasting way.

As Andrea explored and experimented with sex, I maintained a supportive but neutral stance. The therapist should at no time want the client to have sex more than the client herself wants it. This would simply replay the obligation dynamic with different characters. Building on the work Andrea did in identifying the various emotional reasons for having sex, she was able to say no to sex more directly (with less avoidance of Cricket) but also in a kinder and more sympathetic way. It was at this point that our sessions were spaced with longer intervals between appointments. Andrea used therapy to further explore what she liked and didn't like sexually as her new awareness of herself as a sexual being was reinforced.

COMMENTARY

The lesson of Andrea's therapy concerns the vital importance of space. As a sex therapist I often find myself in the role of advocate or cheerleader for good or great or sometimes just adequate sex. Women who come to therapy complaining of low desire don't need a cheerleader for sex. They don't need encouragement to have more or better sex. They do not need to feel that they must live up to the rather masculine ideal of lustful sex. They need a supportive therapeutic relationship in which they can explore their sexual feelings and discover what works (or doesn't) for them in their lives and in their relationships. At times I had to hold myself back from cheering Andrea on, nudging her forward, extolling the virtues of a happy sex life. I had to tell myself that I couldn't want her to have sex more than she wants it. I had to remind myself that it was okay if she decided that she did not want to have a sexual relationship with her partner or anyone else.

In the space of therapy, Andrea was able to sort out messages from her past and confront the shame she felt for the abuse she experienced. She grew to be curious about sex. With permission not to have sex or be sexual, she ultimately found a place for sex in her life. Low sexual desire is a sexual disorder without a clear definition. In essence what constitutes low desire is defined by the client and her partner. The resolution must similarly be defined within the couple. Therapy needs to provide a space in which clients can find their own level of desire.

Sex therapy may be victim to its success and popularity as a brief symptom focused approach to sexual problems. Even though this case had a successful outcome, it took approximately 1 year to reach that point. Andrea had a patient and sympathetic partner who shared her interest in having sex be an expression of love and who, as a psychotherapist, understood that therapy often takes time. Many male partners feel more hurt and upset at the lack of sex. They desperately want to feel wanted and have difficulty tolerating a slow pace of therapy. Many times male partners have wondered whether I, as a woman, can really understand their perspective on sex, their need or desire to be wanted sexually. What I learned from Andrea and Cricket's case was that managing expectations is an important part of therapy. I now tell couples at the outset that therapy is a long process. I share with them both the traditional or male model of sexual desire as well as Basson's model of female sexual desire during the evaluation. I demonstrate throughout therapy an understanding of their divergent perspectives on sex, but I remain resolutely neutral regarding how they will ultimately negotiate their differences. Therapy should give the individual or couple space in which to explore what will inspire their sexual relationship. In cases of low desire, I do not encourage couples to make dates for sex. What I do encourage are dates that give the couple time and space in which sexual desire, interest, or willingness might occur.

Perhaps one of the most important lessons from Andrea's therapy is that given time and space, women will discover the source of their passion. The key in therapy is to facilitate this process while the challenge may be to help the partner provide and maintain that space within the relationship.

Obligation kills desire. Pressure, be it from oneself, one's partner, or one's therapist, will not lead to passion. What does lead to passion will differ across genders and individual clients. It is up to the client to discover it. It is up to the therapist to support the client, and often her partner, through this process.

REFERENCES

Basson, R. (2007). Sexual arousal/desire disorders in women. In S. R. Leiblum (Ed.), *Principles and practice of sex therapy* (4th ed., pp. 25–53). New York: Guilford Press.

Bradford, A., & Meston, C. (2007). Correlates of placebo response in the treatment of sexual dysfunction in women: A preliminary report. *Journal of Sexual Medicine, 4*, 1345–1351.

Hall, K. S. (2004). *Reclaiming your sexual self: How you can bring desire back into your life.* Hoboken, NJ: Wiley.

Joannides, P. (2008). *The guide to getting it on* (6th ed.). Waldport, OR: Goofy Foot Press.

Chapter 5

Confronting Male Hypoactive Sexual Desire Disorder

Secrets, Variant Arousal, and Good-Enough Sex

Barry McCarthy
Alisa Breetz

In this thoughtful chapter, Barry McCarthy and Alisa Breetz observe that dysfunctional, conflictual, or absent sex plays an inordinately negative role in couple intimacy, and that often it is the male partner who decides unilaterally to stop being sexual. Often, the man's lack of desire is secondary to erectile difficulties but at times it is related to undisclosed secrets and shame.

Operating within a cognitive-behavioral framework, McCarthy and Breetz present the case of a man who is avoiding sexual intimacy with his new wife because of an undisclosed sexual fetish—a 20-year history of masturbating to images of women wearing mid-calf boots. The man's reliance on Internet boot fetish sites to arouse and stimulate him is playing havoc with his current marriage to a 37-year-old woman who is eager to become pregnant and greatly distressed about the lack of sexuality in her life.

McCarthy and Breetz discuss their "good-enough sex" approach and use of structured exercises to help recapture desire as well as provide a host of suggestions for relapse prevention.

Barry McCarthy, PhD, is Professor of Psychology at American University and a certified sex and marital therapist who practices individual, couple, and sex therapy at the Washington Psychological Center.

Alisa Breetz, MA, is a graduate student in the clinical psychology doctoral program at American University and has collaborated with Dr. McCarthy on various articles focused on sexual functioning, couple therapy, and sexual trauma.

Clinicians are increasingly reporting that the sexual problem that most subverts couple satisfaction and brings couples to therapy is conflict about sexual desire and extreme sexual avoidance (McCarthy & McCarthy, 2003). Although lay public and media emphasis is on the man's role of pursuing sex and the woman's role of withholding sex, the reality is that when couples stop being sexual (i.e., having sex less than 10 times a year), it is usually the man's decision, made unilaterally and conveyed nonverbally. In understanding, assessing, and treating the problem of male hypoactive sexual desire disorder (HSDD) we advocate a comprehensive, integrative, psychobiosocial approach to male and couple sexuality. In addition, we strongly suggest adopting the "good-enough sex" model, which focuses on valuing a variable, flexible approach to sharing intimacy, pleasure, and eroticism rather than clinging to the traditional male criterion of autonomous erections and perfect intercourse performance.

To date, the greatest attention has been paid to HSDD in women. Basson (2007) has introduced and developed the concept of "responsive sexual desire." This breakthrough therapeutic intervention has destigmatized HSDD and allowed many women to accept the observation that their desire may be more variable and flexible than that of males. Female desire is simply different, neither better nor worse. If sexual desire is defined by the traditional youthful male standard—easy, predictable erections with a focus on sexual frequency and performance—the woman is stuck in the "one down" position. In the traditional model, sexual desire and arousal is a race, and she is the loser.

The comprehensive, integrative, psychobiosocial approach to couple sexuality presents a very different model. We believe that each person is responsible for his or her own desire, arousal, and orgasm. The challenge for couples is to develop their unique couple sexual style and to integrate intimacy and eroticism into their relationship.

The traditional male expectation of easy, predictable erections, total sexual control, and perfect intercourse performance must be confronted as self-defeating.

Traditionally, a man believes that sexual response is autonomous: he can experience desire, arousal, and orgasm without needing anything from his partner. Although this might be characteristic in new relationships, it subverts mature couple sexuality, especially after the ages of 40–50. The new psychobiosocial model views sex as an interpersonal process, not an autonomous one, with the ultimate goal of enhancing relationship satisfaction (Metz & McCarthy, 2007).

The basic paradox in couple sexuality is that sex plays a greater role in overall well-being when it is unhealthy than when it is healthy. Healthy couple sexuality enhances feelings of personal and couple psychological well-being. The paradox is that dysfunctional, conflictual, or nonexistent sexuality has an inordinately powerful negative role, robbing the relationship of intimacy and threatening relationship viability.

MALE HYPOACTIVE SEXUAL DESIRE DISORDER

The majority of men who lack desire are reacting to erectile dysfunction (ED) and/or ejaculatory inhibition (EI). In secondary male HSDD, the man has lost his confidence regarding erections, intercourse, and orgasm. Rather than the healthy cycle of positive anticipation, pleasure-oriented sex, and a regular rhythm of sexual experiences, an unhealthy cycle of anticipatory anxiety, tense, pass–fail intercourse performance, and frustration, embarrassment, and eventually sexual avoidance becomes dominant. Often, sex has become a fearful, embarrassing experience to be avoided. The decision to stop sex is typically made unilaterally by the man and conveyed nonverbally. He thinks, "I don't want to start something I can't finish," and so avoids sensual and sexual touch. By the age of 65, one in three couples has a nonsexual relationship, which increases to two in three couples by age 75 (McKinlay & Feldman, 1994). The cessation of touching and sexuality contributes significantly to a man's view of aging as a loss.

Although pro-erection medications have been viewed as the answer to erection and desire problems, often medical interventions result in a nonsexual relationship because of unrealistic sexual performance expectations.

A less common but more challenging problem is primary male HSDD. Although men with primary HSDD may be sexually functional in a new relationship, the reality is that they often cannot sustain or do not value intimate, interactive couple sex. Typically, the core problem is a sexual secret that they feel must be kept hidden. These secrets may be a variant arousal pattern, a preference for masturbatory sex rather than couple sex (especially using Internet porn), a poorly processed history of sexual trauma that has not been disclosed to the partner, or unverbalized conflict about sexual orientation. This combination of eroticism, secrecy, and shame creates a poisonous and very controlling sexual scenario. Often, the man blames the woman for the sexual problem. She feels confused, frustrated, and rejected, leading to anger and alienation.

CASE EXAMPLE: NICK AND DORA

Nick, age 33, initiated the request for consultation because of increasing marital distress with his second wife, Dora, age 37. She was threatening to leave Nick because their 18-month-old marriage was nonsexual, and had been since before they wed. Dora wanted children and felt great stress about her "biological clock." Nick was extremely distressed at the possibility of being twice divorced before age 35.

Nick's initial request was for individual therapy, but our preferred treatment approach is couple therapy with a four session assessment model. Both partners are seen in the first session, then an individual session is scheduled with each partner to obtain a psychological/relational/sexual history, and finally a couple feedback session for the couple to discuss a therapeutic plan.

The first couple session was quite stressful—clearly, the marriage was in crisis. Dora was extremely confused and agitated about living in a nonsexual marriage. Dora had met Nick at a picnic arranged by married friends who assured her that Nick was committed to both marriage and children. Now Dora felt that Nick had pulled a "bait and switch," and she felt betrayed. Unless their sexual pattern was quickly resolved, Dora threatened to leave the marriage so she could remarry and try to have a child.

Nick presented as the rational, conciliatory spouse who promised this would all work out. His explanation of their problems focused on the stress caused by conflicts about wedding planning, which he blamed primarily on Dora's mother, especially conflicts about religious symbols involved in the wedding ceremony. Nick said he felt badly about the nonsexual state of their marriage, but reassured Dora of his commitment to her and to having children. Nick said that Dora's 15-pound weight gain, pressure to have sex, and accusations that he was a latent homosexual or having an affair were the main barriers to their sexual intimacy.

Their individual sessions were scheduled for the same week, with Nick's session first. The clinician begins the history with the following introduction:

> "I want to understand your psychological, relational, and sexual history both before this marriage and during the marriage. I want to hear both strengths and vulnerabilities. I appreciate your being as forthcoming and blunt as possible. At the end, I'll ask if there is any sensitive or secret material that you do not want shared with your spouse. I will not share it without your permission, but I need to know as much as possible so I can be of help to you in understanding and resolving these problems."

Nick reported beginning masturbation at age 12, and by age 13 he had developed a narrow, controlling fetish pattern involving mid-calf boots. Although he felt shameful about the fetish and compulsive masturbation and had tried multiple times to abstain, the mid-calf boot fetish had dominated his sexuality for the past 20 years. Nick experienced 20–35 orgasms a month, the vast majority involving two Internet boot fetish sites where he charged approximately $700 a month to his credit card. This was a powerful sexual secret he had not shared with Dora or any other woman (including his ex-wife).

Nick said that early in a relationship he would be sexually desirous and functional, but within weeks or months he would develop ejaculatory inhibition. With increased frustration for him and his partner, Nick would avoid intercourse and would revert to masturbatory sex using the fetish site. The clinician labeled Nick the "master of masturbation," which he smilingly acknowledged.

When Nick met Dora he was enthusiastic and hopeful that his pattern would change. He saw Dora as a very attractive and sexually positive woman and he found the first 5 months of his relationship with her sexually rewarding. The cycle ended when Dora insisted on remaining on the birth control pill until they were actually married. Nick wanted a child and felt stymied at what he viewed as Dora's conservatism. He blamed it on her mother, who was a practicing Roman Catholic. Nick had been raised in a nondenominational Christian church but religion played a minimal role in his life.

Once the "magic" of romantic love/passionate sex/idealization was broken, Nick withdrew from Dora sexually and resumed daily masturbation using the mid-calf boot site. They attempted intercourse three times during the honeymoon but Nick was self-conscious, moved to intercourse quickly, and tried to force ejaculation. He focused on his boot fetish fantasies. Dora found the prolonged intercourse physically and emotionally irritating. Nick would "run out of gas" and would either lose his erection or end the sexual encounter. Nick felt frustrated and humiliated and avoided talking with Dora about sex. Outside of sex, however, he continued to value their affectionate relationship.

Past History: Nick

Nick's siblings had established successful marriages and families, although Nick never discussed sexual issues with them. He was emotionally closer to his mother, who had struggled financially following the divorce from Nick's father. His father had a history of extramarital affairs, and a year after the divorce he married the woman with whom he was having an affair. However within 2 years his father was divorced again. Nick prided himself on not having affairs and was shocked by the clinician's question of whether he viewed the fetish as a type of affair. Nick had never thought of the fetish as a secret sexual life, equivalent to an affair.

As he talked about Dora and his fear that she would leave him, it was clear that Nick was in great distress. While Nick desperately wanted a successful marriage and family, he felt controlled by his secret sexual life. Nick wanted Dora's love and acceptance, but was afraid to share his sexual dilemma with her.

Typically, at the conclusion of the individual history, several open-ended questions are asked:

1. "What else should I know about you psychologically, relationally, or sexually?"
2. "As you look back on your entire life, what was the most negative, confusing, guilt-inducing, or traumatic thing that ever happened to you?"

3. "Is there anything you want to red-flag and not have me share with your spouse?"
4. "Is there anything you want to ask or check out with me?"

Nick said that he really wanted to remain married and have children with Dora. His secret (and expensive) fetish was the major negative reality of his life, but he was afraid to share it because of Dora's possible reaction. The clinician actively lobbied Nick to disclose his secret since the best time to share sensitive material is during the couple feedback session. The clinician repeated the 12-step program mantra: "You are only as sick as your secrets."

Nick also agreed to attend his first meeting of the 12-step fellowship Sex Addicts Anonymous (SAA). Receiving acceptance and support from group members, especially through a relationship with a sponsor, is of great value in reducing stigma and shame as well as improving accountability with respect to compulsive/addictive behavior.

Past History: Dora

Earlier in her life, Dora saw herself as a smart, attractive woman who liked men and sex, but the stress of dating had truly worn her down. She had initially felt optimistic about Nick, but her disappointment in the lack of sex was profound and her fears of never having a family overwhelming. Dora felt unattractive and nonsexual and for the first time in her adult life had ceased masturbating. Men flirted with her and she reported two invitations to have an affair but decided not to act on these invitations unless she was officially separated. However, awareness of these opportunities made the option of a separation more compelling.

Dora believed that Nick had a sexual secret—either that he was homosexual or having an affair with another woman. She felt pressured from her individual therapist to move on with her life since she was 37. The worst obstacle in Dora's life was the pattern of being disappointed and let down by men—her father, boyfriends, and now Nick. Dora felt depressed and was herself experiencing low desire.

Couple Feedback Session

The 90-minute couple feedback session is the core intervention in this therapeutic model. As with the vast majority of couples, the clinician had received permission to share sensitive and secret material in a therapeutic manner.

The feedback session has three goals: (1) to develop a genuinely new individual and couple narrative regarding intimacy and sexuality, (2) to agree on a therapeutic plan and contract, and (3) to assign a psychosexual skill exercise to begin to address desire issues.

The feedback started with enumerating Nick's personal and sexual strengths: He was a competent, well-intentioned male who loved Dora and wanted a successful marriage and family; he could experience desire, arousal, and orgasm; he was finally willing to face difficult sexual issues; he was an empathic problem solver.

Clearly, Nick's greatest vulnerability was the secret, shameful boot fetish. Its power was demonstrated by normally frugal Nick spending a great deal of money on Internet sex, by his reluctance to enlist Dora as his intimate ally (instead further alienating her by raising false issues about her weight and the mother-in-law's role), and by his lack of comfort and confidence with intimate, interactive sex.

The clinician gave Nick a chance to change, edit, or add to the narrative, but Nick said it was "spot on." The clinician asked Dora whether she needed to clarify any information or perceptions about Nick's sexual narrative. Dora wanted to be sure she had the whole story and that there was not an affair or any other emotional or sexual secret which would be revealed later. Throughout this feedback session an important therapeutic strategy was to avoid strong negative emotions.

The same process was repeated for Dora's narrative with Nick listening. Dora was surprised at the accuracy of her narrative, especially how rejected and demoralized she felt. Dora felt validated by the recital of her personal, relational, and sexual strengths. Nick commented on how sad he felt about Dora's feelings of depression, sexual rejection, and diminished desire.

The second phase of the feedback session involves outlining the therapeutic focus and contract—a 6-month good-faith effort to build a new couple sexual style, to confront the sexual poison of a secret fetish life, and to affirm marital vitality by having a planned, wanted child. It was clear to the clinician that this would be a daunting task but, if Nick and Dora stayed focused and motivated, a realizable one.

The third phase was a psychosexual trust exercise, which focused on developing a "trust position." The couple are presented with several examples of physical positions (e.g., she puts her head on his chest and listens to his heartbeat; they lie together in a spoon position and verbally acknowledged feeling cared for and secure). In the privacy of their home, they try out and find one position where they feel comfortable, connected, and safe. In the case of Nick and Dora, we started with trust because it addressed a core issue and was likely to be successfully implemented. In addition, Nick agreed to find someone from the SAA group who was able to put a "block" on the fetish sites.

At the beginning of the weekly couple sex therapy session, Dora reported that the trust exercise had been powerfully energizing for her in physically reconnecting with Nick for the first time since their marriage. The computer blocking program had been successfully installed and Dora held the code. Nick joked that money would be better spent on therapy than compulsive cybersex.

The next psychosexual skill technique involved a comfort exercise to share pleasure and intimate feelings and heighten the erotic experience. The exercise is done in the privacy of their home. They experiment with touching inside and outside the bedroom; clothed, semiclothed, or nude; being silent or mixing talking and touching; taking turns or doing mutual touch to establish receptivity and responsivity to touch scenarios and techniques. As part of the comfort exercise there was a prohibition on Nick trying to force orgasm and turning away from Dora when he failed. Not surprisingly, Dora found the experience more fulfilling than Nick. Dora transitioned to the trust position after less than 5 minutes of intercourse when she sensed that sexual intercourse was no longer pleasurable or involving for Nick. He affirmed her perception, and this helped him see Dora as his intimate sexual friend rather than someone to perform for so she wouldn't abandon him. In that same week, Dora asked Nick to hold her while she pleasured herself to orgasm. This was very sexually arousing for Nick, who was aroused by her arousal and experienced her sexual response as a good thing rather than as pressure to match her response.

During the next therapy session, they had an emotional discussion over the importance of Nick sharing his struggles with sexual compulsivity. The hardest thing for Nick to accept was that couple sex could not have the extreme intensity of fetish sex, although it could be more genuine and satisfying.

The next psychosexual skill exercise was an "attraction" exercise to identify what Nick genuinely found attractive (physically, emotionally, sexually, and interpersonally) about Dora. This exercise had a powerful energizing effect on Dora and helped to undue the damage his defensive attacks on her weight and attractiveness had caused. Nick also requested that (1) Dora be open to his erotic stimulation because her arousal was arousing for him, (2) they shop together at Victoria's Secret for sexy clothing, (3) she engage in multiple stimulation during intercourse (e.g., being open to receiving breast stimulation and giving testicle stimulation). In addition, Nick's requests assured Dora that he wanted and needed her as his erotic partner.

Building bridges to desire is a couple task. Most helpful for Nick and Dora was to have "his," "hers," and "our" bridges to sexual desire. Dora needed to regain her "sexual voice" and to be receptive and responsive to both partner-interaction and self-entrancement arousal. This in turn facilitated Nick's sexual desire and response. Dora's openness to engaging in multiple stimulation during intercourse was particularly valuable. In addition, Dora accepted Nick using self-stimulation during erotic, nonintercourse sex. Her use of sexy clothing (a variation of role enactment arousal) was not a substitute for the mid-calf boot fetish, but a different bridge to desire and an erotic stimulus. Dora's enthusiasm in pleasuring and eroticism allowed Nick to "piggy-back" his arousal on hers. The clinician emphasized the importance of being both intimate and erotic friends rather than competitors for ease and rapidity of sexual response.

Confronting Variant Arousal

Addressing Nick's variant arousal pattern was challenging. Although some clinicians advocate the woman accepting the man's variant arousal and integrating it into their couple sexual style, we believe that this is not a genuine option for the majority of men with a secret sexual life. The narrowness and rigidity of fetish sex is such that it does not integrate into couple intimacy and eroticism. The analogy that Nick found most helpful was that the mid-calf boot fetish was like "sexual heroin." The erotic charge from the fetish was extraordinarily powerful and had been reinforced by tens of thousands of Internet/masturbatory orgasms. The combination of eroticism, secrecy, and shame was as compelling as heroin and ultimately just as destructive to Nick's life, especially his marriage and hope for a family. Nick's commitment to totally abstaining from the fetish was not caused by moralistic reasoning, but by the understanding that it would control and poison not only his life but their couple relationship as well. Good intentions were not enough. Nick needed to use all his resources, including regular attendance at SAA meetings, a relationship with a sponsor, maintaining the computer block on fetish sites, developing an intimate and erotic couple sexual style, couple sex therapy, and checking in monthly with Dora to ensure there was no regression to a secret sexual life (i.e., maintaining transparency).

Variant arousal is truly an intimacy disorder. While couple sexuality is necessary, it is not sufficient for overcoming a long-standing variant arousal pattern. Both Dora and Nick needed to be aware that even the healthiest couple sexuality would not be enough to break the cycle of sexual compulsivity.

In subsequent couple sessions at least 10 minutes were devoted to discussing Nick's compulsive sexual behavior. For most men, sexually compulsive behavior is a chronic issue. For a minority of men, the fetish loses its power once the secrecy is confronted and awareness of the harmful effects of compulsive sex become clear. Unfortunately, Nick needed to consistently monitor the fetish to prevent a relapse into his secret world. Nick struggled with his "sexual demon." The strength of his sexual urges to act out the fetish arousal was quite distinct from marital and sexual satisfaction. Originally, Dora hoped that love, a renewed marital commitment, and a satisfying sex life would be enough to change the variant arousal pattern. It was a sobering realization for both Nick and Dora to accept that this was a separate issue that required vigilance and monitoring.

Sexual Desire and Conception

Perhaps the most difficult, but crucial, discussion occurred during the ninth therapy session. Nick and Dora had resumed intercourse, and Dora was not using birth control. The question was whether they felt confident enough of their marital and sexual commitment to have a planned, wanted baby.

The issue for Dora was whether a baby would cement their marital bond or destabilize marital sex and reignite Nick's sexual compulsivity. As they discussed these complex issues, the clinician took the role of facilitater, helping the couple make a wise decision, rather than being the decision maker. It was crucial that Dora believe Nick had her best interests in mind and that he would not do anything to intentionally undermine her or their marital bond. Nick was able to make that commitment. Although there could be "lapses"—incidents of masturbating to images of the boot fetish or even using Internet stimuli—Nick was committed to transparency, to enhancing marital sexuality, and to not allowing his lapse to become a relapse to a secret sexual life.

Nick assured Dora he would not let her become pregnant and then abandon the marriage. She assured him of her love and of the value she placed on both marriage and family. Nick's other major concern was that Dora would never truly forgive him for his past behavior. Dora wanted a marriage with Nick where they maintained a secure attachment through good and bad times, including couple sexual issues and compulsive sexuality.

Intercourse with the hope and intention of becoming pregnant is an aphrodisiac for most couples. It certainly was for Nick and Dora. They committed to having intercourse two to three times during the week with the greatest probability of fertility. Much to Nick's surprise, the impetus of pregnancy enhanced his sexual desire. Initiating intercourse only at high levels of arousal and using multiple stimulation and erotic fantasies (but not the boot fetish) as an orgasm trigger resulted in pleasurable, functional intercourse and intravaginal ejaculation. Much to Dora's surprise she became pregnant within 3 months.

Sessions were now scheduled biweekly in order to maintain the gains they had made. On the weeks when we did not meet, Nick and Dora were encouraged to preserve the time for themselves in order to talk, have a sexual date, go for a walk, have lunch, engage in a psychosexual skill exercise, or simply be with each other. An advantage of couple time is that it facilitates being together without the distractions of work, chores, and other agendas.

The more variable and flexible couple sexuality is, the less likelihood of relapse. Nick and Dora needed to refine their initiation patterns, maintain affectionate touch both inside and outside of the bedroom (while recognizing that not all touch could or should lead to intercourse), develop and refine erotic scenarios and techniques, view intercourse as a natural continuation of the pleasuring/eroticism process (rather than as a pass–fail performance test), integrate afterplay scenarios and techniques that promote bonding and satisfaction, and accept the varied roles and meanings of couple sexuality (as a shared pleasure, a means of expressing loving feelings, a tension reducer to alleviate stress, a "port in the storm," one-way sex to soothe a disappointment, couple sex to breach an argument or feelings of alienation, a way to reaffirm attraction and vitality).

An Individualized Relapse Prevention Plan

In an individualized relapse prevention plan it is crucial that the couple realize that sexual desire must be consistently nurtured. Otherwise, a high rate of relapse is likely. Individually and together the couple needs to build anticipation and bridges to desire, and integrate intimacy and eroticism into their lives and marriage. Just as important, they need to monitor "traps" that can subvert and "poisons" that can kill desire.

Before formal treatment was terminated, Nick and Dora received a handout of 10 relapse prevention strategies/techniques (Metz & McCarthy, 2004), which can be found in Table 5.1. They were asked to choose 2 to 4 that were personally relevant. Since they were expecting a baby, one technique was an agreement that at least one weekend a year they would go away as a couple without the baby. Fortunately, Dora's parents and sister indicated they would be pleased to babysit for a night, weekend, or even a week.

The other major relapse prevention technique agreed upon was to plan a sexual date with a prohibition on intercourse once every 6 weeks. This was particularly important for Dora, who strongly valued the role of playfulness in couple sexuality. Dora found it easier than Nick to accept that intimate, interactive couple sex was not as erotically powerful as the old fetish pattern. As the clinician said, "Don't compare apples and oranges," but instead realize that your new sexual style fits your life and marriage.

There were two important structural factors in their relapse prevention program. First, they scheduled 6-month follow-up sessions over a 2-year period. At each session, the couple checked in on the state of intimacy and sexuality, reviewed progress on reaching the goal for the previous 6 months, and set an enhancement goal for the next 6 months. The goal could be something small, such as trying a new sensual lotion or a different sequence of pleasuring/eroticism, or something big, such as experimenting with a role enactment scenario or going away for the weekend to enhance their intimate and erotic connection.

A second major structural factor in relapse prevention is the use of a "booster session." If they had gone 2 weeks without a significant sexual encounter, the higher-desire partner (in this case, Dora) agreed to initiate sex. If that was not successful, on the third week the other partner (Nick) agreed to initiate. If they had gone a month without a significant sexual encounter, they called for a booster therapy session.

TABLE 5.1. Relapse Prevention Strategies and Guidelines

1. Set aside quality couple time and discuss what you need to do individually and as a couple to maintain a satisfying, intimate relationship.

2. Every 6 months have a formal follow-up meeting either by yourselves or with a therapist to ensure that you remain aware and do not slip back into unhealthy sexual attitudes, behaviors, or feelings. Set individual and couple goals for the next 6 months.

3. Every 4–8 weeks plan a sensual pleasuring session or a playful erotic session where you have a prohibition on intercourse. This allows you to experiment with new sensual stimuli (alternative pleasuring position, body lotion, or new setting) or a playful, erotic scenario (being sexual in the shower, a different oral sex position or sequence, one-way rather than mutual sex). This reminds you to value sharing pleasure rather than intercourse performance and to develop a broad-based, flexible sexual relationship.

4. Five to 15% of sexual experiences are dissatisfying or dysfunctional. That is normal, not a reason to panic or feel like a failure. Maintaining positive, realistic expectations about marital sexuality is a major resource.

5. Accept occasional lapses, but do not allow a lapse to become a relapse. Treat a dysfunctional sexual experience as a normal variation, a mistake to learn from. You are a sexual couple, not a perfectly functioning sex machine. Whether once every 10 times, once a month, or once a year, you will have a lapse (dysfunctional or dissatisfying sex). You can laugh or shrug off the experience and make a date in the next 1 to 3 days when you have the time and energy for an intimate, pleasurable, erotic experience. The importance of setting aside quality time, especially intimacy dates and a weekend away without children, cannot be emphasized enough. Couples report better sex on vacations, validating the importance of getting away, even if only for an afternoon.

6. There is not "one right way" to be sexual. Each couple develops their own unique style of initiation, pleasuring, erotic scenarios and techniques, intercourse, and afterplay. Rather than treating your couple sexual style with benign neglect, be open to modifying or adding something new or special each year.

7. "Good-enough sex" has a range from disappointing to great. The single most important technique in relapse prevention is to accept and not overreact to experiences which are mediocre, dissatisfying, or dysfunctional. Take pride in having an accepting and resilient couple sexual style.

8. Develop a range of intimate, pleasurable, and erotic ways to connect, reconnect, and maintain connection. These include five "gears" (dimensions) of touch:
   a. Affectionate touch (clothes on): kissing, hand-holding, hugs
   b. Nongenital sensual touch (clothed, semiclothed, or nude): massage (excluding genitals), cuddling on the couch, touching before going to sleep or on awakening
   c. Playful touch (semiclothed or nude): mixing nongenital and genital touch, dancing together, touching while showering or bathing, "making out" on the couch
   d. Erotic, nonintercourse touch: using manual, oral, rubbing, or vibrator stimulation to high arousal and/or orgasm for one or both partners
   e. Intercourse: sensuality, playfulness, eroticism naturally flow into intercourse. The more ways to maintain an intimate sexual connection, the easier to avoid relapse.

TABLE 5.1. (continued)

9. Saturate each other with multidimensional touch.

10. Keep your sexual relationship vital. Continue to make sexual requests and be open to exploring erotic scenarios. The importance of maintaining a sexual relationship that serves a 15–20% role of energizing your marital bond and facilitating special feelings of desirability and satisfaction cannot be overemphasized. Couples who share intimacy, nondemand pleasuring, erotic scenarios and techniques, and planned as well as spontaneous sexual encounters have a variable, flexible sexual relationship. This is a major antidote to relapse.

The focus of the session was to identify the "message" behind the sexual avoidance and to problem-solve how to break the avoidance cycle. Although we value supportive, clothes-on affectionate touch (holding hands, hugging, kissing) as a safe, secure form of connection, this is not sexual touch. Sensual, playful, erotic, nonintercourse, as well as intercourse, are all dimensions of healthy couple sexuality. The challenge for Nick and Dora was to use variable, flexible sensual and sexual touch to stay connected. In addition, they learned to value a "good-enough sex" approach to couple sexuality rather than cling to the pass–fail criterion of perfect intercourse performance.

COMMENTARY

Nick and Dora successfully confronted two poisons—a nonsexual marriage and Nick's secret fetish world. Formal treatment involved nine weekly sessions, eight biweekly sessions, one booster session, and three 6-month follow-up sessions. At the last follow-up, they were busy parenting a 19-month-old son and Dora was 2 months pregnant with their second child.

Nick continued his involvement with the SAA fellowship, attending weekly meetings, and continued the monthly check-in process with Dora. Both rated marital satisfaction in the A– range; Dora rated sexual satisfaction in the B+ range, while Nick rated it as a B. Nick's task was to accept himself and commitment to marital and sexual intimacy as the very best he could do and be. Nick felt accepted and loved by Dora, but also felt somewhat frustrated with the fact that sex with Dora was not more erotically fulfilling. Nick wanted to be an especially good sexual educator for his son so that he did not have to go through the pain of harboring a secret, variant arousal pattern.

Couple sex therapy for low desire is an excellent example of the need for an integrative, comprehensive, psychobiosocial model for assessment, treatment, and relapse prevention. The clinician as well as each individual and the couple are urged to use all relevant resources to address the complex, multidimensional issues characteristic of HSDD.

Psychologically, the keys to desire are positive anticipation and a sense of deserving. Biologically, it is crucial to address hormonal and medical deficits, as well as illness, the side effects of medications, and poor health habits. Medical resources are not stand-alone interventions, but rather must be integrated into the couple style of intimacy, pleasuring, and eroticism. Relationally, the partner is viewed as an intimate and erotic friend.

The role of psychosexual skills is of particular importance in developing and maintaining sexual desire. Our cultural view of desire and sexual performance holds that it is simple and "natural." In reality, the challenge for both individuals and couples is to integrate intimacy and eroticism into their ongoing relationship after the initial charge of romantic love/passionate sex/idealization has dissipated. This requires that the woman value her "sexual voice" and that the man learn to value intimacy and nondemand pleasuring. Both partners need to integrate these into their sexual life together.

Finally, couples must have positive, realistic sexual expectations. Accepting that couple sexuality is inherently variable and flexible can be empowering rather than anxiety provoking or discouraging. Sexual desire can be facilitated and enhanced or it can be subverted and poisoned. The "good-enough sex" model promotes sexual desire for men, women, and couples (McCarthy & Metz, 2008).

REFERENCES

Basson, R. (2007). Sexual desire/arousal disorder in women. In S. Leiblum (Ed.). *Principles and practice of sex therapy* (4th ed., pp 25–53). New York: Guilford Press.

McCarthy, B., & McCarthy, E. (2003). *Rekindling desire: A step-by-step program to help low-sex and no-sex marriages*. New York: Brunner/Routledge.

McCarthy, B., & Metz, M. (2008). *Men's sexual health: Fitness for satisfying sex*. New York: Routledge.

McKinlay, J., & Feldman, H. (1994). Age-related variation in sexual activity and interest in normal men. In A. Rossi (Ed.), *Sexuality across the life course* (pp. 261–285). Chicago: University of Chicago Press.

Metz, M., & McCarthy, B. (2004). *Coping with erectile dysfunction: How to regain confidence and enjoy great sex.* Oakland, CA: New Harbinger.

Metz, M., & McCarthy, B. (2007). The good-enough sex model for couple sexual satisfaction. *Sexual and Relationship Therapy, 22*(3), 351–362.

Chapter 6

"Desire Disorders" or Opportunities for Optimal Erotic Intimacy?

Peggy J. Kleinplatz

Aim at heaven and you will get Earth thrown in. Aim at
Earth and you get neither.

—C. S. Lewis

In this chapter, Peggy J. Kleinplatz artfully illustrates how Experiential Psychotherapy and her own unique views of the opportunities afforded by sexuality are used to deal with desire complaints. She observes that although her clinical approach emphasizes personality growth and discovery (in the presence of the partner), sexual problems are usually resolved as well.

One of the significant aspects of therapy is the focus on achieving erotic intimacy or what Kleinplatz describes as the "inter-penetration of the partners, including their wishes, hopes, desires, fantasies, dreams, and fears via sexuality" so that each may have an entry into their partner's inner world. Optimal sexuality—what makes sexuality memorable—involves being fully present, authentic, vulnerable, intensely connected with the partner, and emotionally willing to take risks during sex. It is this subjective and erotic experience that is valued as a therapeutic goal over any objective indice of "normative" sexuality, such as increasing sexual frequency.

In her clinical illustration, Kleinplatz describes several palpable moments when Mrs. Carter identifies a powerful, often painful emotion associated with a past event and gives expression both to the feeling and a more empowered, assertive response. By translating this response to her everyday world and interactions, Mrs. Carter is able to access and experience sex that is worth desiring. Although the therapy is relatively brief, the impact is long-lasting.

Peggy J. Kleinplatz, PhD, is Associate Professor in the Faculty of Medicine and Clinical Professor in the School of Psychology, University of Ottawa, in Ottawa, Canada. Her clinical and research work focuses on optimal sexuality, eroticism, and transformation, with a particular interest in the elderly, sexual minorities, and other marginalized populations.

OVERVIEW OF PROBLEMS OF SEXUAL DESIRE

Desire problems are the most common sexual problems seen in my practice. Some months they comprise a higher proportion of the cases than all other sexual problems combined. Often I think that almost all sexual problems are based in conflict over too much sex, too little sex, or the "wrong" kinds of sex. The frequent comment "If I never had sex again I wouldn't miss it" inevitably leads me to question why this individual is in my office and why now.

Frequently, individuals with low desire say that they have never had sexual desire or at least not much desire. However, a little probing often reveals that if they do not recall having desire for "sex" as they have come to define it, they may recall incidents of very high arousal and excitement and desire in the past. However, what they have come to label as "sex" now is not worth wanting.

Complaints typically come from the higher-desire partner. Even when the lower desire client reports freely, "I'm the one who needs treatment. I've come across this before. It's me. It's why my other relationships have ended and I don't want this one (or the next one) to end because of my problem, too" I am not clear as to the nature of the problem. Sometimes low desire is only evidence of good judgment.

Two types of considerations/conceptualization govern my work with clients referred for treatment of sexual desire disorders: One comes from the experiential model of personality and psychotherapy (Mahrer, 1978, 1996, 2002; Mahrer & Boulet, 2001); the other comes from sexology and in particular, my own approach to eroticism and optimal sexuality (Kleinplatz, 1992, 1996, 2004, 2006; Kleinplatz & Krippner, 2005; Kleinplatz & Ménard, 2007). The methods and goals that emerge from these ways of thinking meld nicely in dealing with low desire (and other sexual concerns) in therapy. Both ways of thinking lead me to focus less on the nature of desire disorders and to concentrate instead on how the individuals involved might grow and how their sex lives might be closer to optimal.

Experiential Psychotherapy* (Mahrer, 1996) is unique, brings about fundamental change relatively quickly, and may seem intimidating to those unfamiliar with this approach. The goal of therapy is not to ameliorate the symptom but to use the presenting problem as an opportunity for growth. Change is brought about by going within rather than attempting to achieve some externally imposed set of goals, whether from the therapist or the higher-desire spouse. Working with moments of peak experiencing helps to bring about substantive personality change. Thus, in Experiential Psychotherapy one never sets out to treat (the symptoms of) sexual (or other) disorders. However, often the personality changes that occur during the course of therapy are so substantial that sexual disorders seem to be "cured" nonetheless (Kleinplatz, 1998, 1999, 2004, 2007).

The methods of Experiential Psychotherapy differ markedly from those of conventional sex therapy. Each session includes four steps (Mahrer 1996): The initial step involves entering into a moment of strong feeling in order to find and access some deeper way of being within the individual. During the second step, the client welcomes this new experiencing by beginning to identify it and receive it, for example, by attending to the bodily sensations that accompany the emerging way of being. During the third step, the client returns to earlier life events during which this inner experiencing could have and should have been present, although it has not generally been available in many years. The client returns to the past and lives as the newly accessed deeper experiencing, giving voice and expression to the way of being that he or she might have been and can now choose to become. In the final step, the client, still in the office, tries out and rehearses the newly revived inner way of being in prospective new opportunities in the "real" postsession world. Homework is usually generated by the "new" client, who plans to carry on being the person he or she might have been after conclusion of the session.

Although Experiential Psychotherapy was designed to be used in individual therapy, it offers a particular advantage in dealing with sexual problems in couple therapy (Kleinplatz, 1999, 2007). It is a

---

*Experiential Psychotherapy as described by Mahrer (1996) is usually capitalized to distinguish this model of psychotherapy from the rather large family of other experiential approaches to psychotherapy.

truism in couple therapy that changes to one of the individuals creates a threat to the couple system. One advantage of this method is that the partner's presence helps make change safer for the couple—being a witness to the therapy process may increase respect for the partner's courage, thereby enhancing relationship intimacy. The Experiential models of personality change and psychotherapy emphasize optimal ways of being and behaving (Mahrer, 1996, 2008a, 2008b). There is something profoundly exciting for both parties when they begin to envision a relationship that is more than merely free of problems but one in which sex begins to soar—or more correctly, when the participants begin to glimpse how it might feel to be utterly alive and engaged in each other's embrace. Perhaps most fundamentally, Experiential Psychotherapy places a primacy on subjective experience over objective indices of behavior, such as sexual functioning, performance, and frequency.

Similarly, a focus on optimal sexuality and eroticism in sex therapy shifts the emphasis from how often couples engage in sex to whether or not the sex they habitually engage in is worth wanting. The assumption here is that a lot of cases of low desire stem from unfulfilling sex. The conflation of frequency counts with assessments of pleasure, joy, and delight makes it too easy to get sidetracked into recording progress in terms of how often the couple has sex, which can eclipse attention to the quality of the sex.

From this vantage point, the definition of "sex" offered by many people referred for treatment of low desire is so narrow as to preclude desire. The definition tends to feature tension relief, intercourse, and orgasm. If "sex" is to be a few perfunctory moments of "foreplay" followed by penetration so as to get "sex" over with as quickly as possible, it is hard to imagine why anyone would want it, not to mention why anyone would put up with such uninspired, bland, lackluster, and, indeed, undesirable sex. Even worse, if the chief motive for going through the motions is to be able to count this event as having "done it" in order to prevent interpersonal conflict—as in, "if I don't 'do it' he [or she] gets grumpy"—then sex is bound to be empty, if not outright laden with resentment. It is even more disturbing that either partner would choose to endure such a chore in the name of peace or, more accurately, to buy some temporary relational détente.

In this clinical approach, the focus is not on acts or techniques or performance but on erotic intimacy. By erotic intimacy, I am referring to the knowing interpenetration of the partners, including their wishes, hopes, desires, fantasies, dreams, and fears, via sexuality.

Eroticism is about the intent to arouse and to heighten that arousal for the sheer joy of it and for the sake of having an entry point into the partner's inner world (Kleinplatz, 1992, 1996, 2006). It is about allowing the vulnerability that one or both partners experience in this endeavor to be exposed in the hope that whatever is discovered will be accepted, valued, cherished, and regarded as precious. Eroticism can potentially go beyond the sensory and may involve the entire range of intrapsychic and interpersonal elements (Kleinplatz, 1992, 1996). In an erotic encounter, the lover feels valued knowing that his/her partner is interested enough in him or her as an erotic being to enjoy the process of attempting to provide erotic fulfilment rather than merely aiming for orgasm. The passion of eroticism may perhaps be most profound when both partners sense they are touching one another's deeper, inner, hidden selves, rather than only their bodies. The sense of intimacy that comes from this sort of carnal knowledge, used here deliberately as a descriptor of a profound, shared state rather than as a euphemism for "having sex," is the essence of eroticism.

Recently my research team has been investigating empirically the phenomenon of optimal sexuality among key informants, that is, individuals who have experienced optimal sexuality, primarily in relationships of 25 years or more. Our findings have shown that, indeed, there are aspects of extraordinary sex reported almost universally among individuals despite different educational and socioeconomic backgrounds and diverse sexual histories. These qualities include being fully present, authentic, vulnerable, intensely connected with the partner, and taking emotional risks during sex (Kleinplatz & Ménard, 2007; Kleinplatz et al., 2009).

Putting the clinical and research pieces together, whatever kind of sex works for two (or more) individuals will be more enticing if the partners are alive, embodied and integrated within themselves and absorbed in and engaged with one another in the moment. The particulars will be unique to each individual; in fact, that is what makes sex so erotic—that each encounter involves two sets of sexual arousal patterns and accompanying meanings, each as distinctive as fingerprints. However, the commonality is that the individuals choose to go outside the boundaries of conventional sex scripts and knowingly reveal themselves, being emotionally naked together with awareness of the risks engendered in this endeavor.

In summary, where these complementary approaches meet is in privileging subjective experience over objective indices of behavior and individual uniqueness over normative sexuality and in the assumption that in order for "sex" (whatever that entails) to be desirable, it will have to be deeply engaging to the individuals in question.

Here is where this approach to thinking about people and change in psychotherapy intertwines with the role of eroticism in dealing with low desire: The goals of therapy from the vantage points of Experiential Psychotherapy and promoting optimal sexuality involve making the relationship *just* safe enough for the partners to be vulnerable, authentic, and engaged together. Sharing in erotic intimacy presupposes two individuals capable of being and choosing to be alive in their skin together.

Challenging Conventional Assumptions

The challenges in cases of low desire or sexual desire discrepancy are posed primarily by the unspoken assumptions about sexuality held by the general public (and sometimes within the field of sex therapy) and reinforced by the media. These assumptions include the following: the problem is the quantity of sex rather than the quality; sex is equated with intercourse (in heterosexual couples); low desire is viewed as a problem to be treated rather than a message calling for attention to something deeper in the individual and/or the couple, or an opportunity for growth; and the goal of treatment is to increase sexual frequency.

Hollywood images set couples up for the bizarre belief that everyone should want "sex" whenever it is available regardless of meaning and context. Patients are thus often in the position of choosing to compromise between what looks easy on the screen but is unattainable and what they have known as arduous and dull but should implicitly be wanted and engaged in for the sake of the relationship.

In addition, gender role norms work to everyone's disadvantage; the notion that men and women are essentially and fundamentally different leads to an awful lot of condescension and resentment. Feelings of being unwanted are often buried or are expressed as anger rather than sorrow or hurt.

CASE EXAMPLE: KAREN AND MARK CARTER

The case illustration presented here is a representative and relatively ordinary case, similar to the ones I see routinely in my practice.

Karen Carter had been in therapy previously for treatment of depression, low self-esteem, and body-image problems and was referred to me for treatment of low desire. Previous therapy 2 years before seemed to manage the symptoms of depression but did not result in broader change. She had been using oral contraceptives for 12 years except when trying to conceive. Mrs. Carter is in good health and not on any medications. An IUD is used for birth control.

There were a total of seven therapy sessions in addition to one follow-up session 6 months later and a final session at the 18-month mark. The first session involved meeting with Mrs. Carter alone, and all the subsequent sessions included Mr. and Mrs. Carter in couple therapy. No matter who the identified patient is, whoever is bothered by the problem really ought to be present if therapy is to be most effective.

Mr. and Mrs. Carter have been together since their late teens and have never had sexual partners other than each other. "We were so young and so nervous when we started." They married almost 20 years ago and are now in their early 40s. They have three children ranging in age from 9 to 17 years old. They report having "a really good relationship" with "much love." However, Mrs. Carter feels no desire for sex: "It's not as if I feel a void. I don't think about it. I don't dream about it. It's not that I'm not attracted to him. I find him very attractive. I just have no desire. It's been this way for many years ... almost from the beginning ... from when we started having sex."

The couple had been having sex once a month for at least 10 years. Prior to that, sex occurred roughly once per week. Since their marriage, there had never been enough sexual activity for Mr. Carter, but at least during the years when they were trying to have children, Mrs. Carter put in her fair share of the effort and would initiate occasionally. After their youngest daughter was born, the decrease in sexual frequency was gradual but noticeable over time. Mr. Carter commented, "This is very hard because I find her extremely attractive." Mrs. Carter responded, "Well, you know I try for a few weeks at a time ... and then I slip." Mr. Carter replied, "It makes me feel that I'm not a priority for her ... I care very much about her satisfaction. I try to be a good lover. I wish she enjoyed it is much as I do, so she'd look forward to it ... I'm seeking more than physical fulfillment."

Over the years Mr. Carter had coped by retreating from all physical contact, then in moments of desperation would return to initiating sex with Mrs. Carter. When he observed her "giving in" with a marked lack of enthusiasm, he would retreat again, with increasingly longer intervals without sexual or other physical intimacy. Mr. Carter no longer initiates because he knows his wife will say "yes" but "for [what he considers] the wrong reasons."

Mrs. Carter has no desire to initiate. "But I get emotional fulfillment from making him happy." He counters, "I get turned off by not having her want sex per se. I perceive her as feeling it's more of a 'have to.'"

When I inquired as to what brought them into therapy at this time, Mr. Carter reported that he had been in a serious car accident 1 year earlier and had been unable to engage in intercourse temporarily. This scare had been a wake-up call for him and created a sense of urgency about a future without sex. Finally, Mr. Carter had reached the point where one day a few months earlier he had simply stopped in mid-thrust and rolled away from his wife. "I just stopped and confronted her that I couldn't go on this way." Thereafter he became nonresponsive and nonaffectionate and "that led to our finally discussing the problem."

In using the Experiential approach, formal history taking is rare. However, enough data about the past, present, and especially the future emerge nonetheless.

Past History

Mrs. Carter's parents separated when she was 6 years old. After her father left, she had no further contact with him until adulthood. In previous therapy she had identified abandonment issues but dealt with them with limited success. Her mother did not have the resources, financially or emotionally, to raise her alone, so she was raised by both her mother and her grandmother in a home with many rules (e.g., eat this, do not wear that) and few boundaries (e.g., no privacy in bedrooms or the bathroom). "My grandmother would walk in while I was in the shower to hurry me up until I was 15." She had little ownership of her body in that environment, although she did try: "I would get caught breaking every single rule." There was no history of sexual abuse. Messages about sexuality were mixed. "I hit puberty early and was teased a lot. I became very self-conscious. Mom would always say, 'If you've got it flaunt it' but I never did. *My mother* did and I thought it was gross." Indeed, Karen's resulting, lifelong self-consciousness and inhibitions about her voluptuous figure would later become an issue in therapy. Mrs. Carter began self-stimulating at 12 or 13 and was "caught" by her grandmother who told the rest of the family: "They found it funny. Nothing was sacred in that house. Nothing was private . . . .so I stopped."

Mr. Carter grew up in a traditional nuclear family with two loving but overprotective parents. They never spoke about sex and he learned considerably from their silence. He was taught to always be a gentleman, but could only surmise what this meant in a highly sex-negative environment. He tried to be respectful of women but was not clear on the extent to which his reticence was in deference to their delicate sensibilities versus his own need to play it safe and be inoffensive.

When Mark and Karen began dating, he waited almost a year to first initiate intercourse. "I went very slowly with her. I wanted to make her feel comfortable." Mrs. Carter added, "There was a lot of making out and [to her surprise] several months before we had oral sex." As he said, "I wanted it to come from her. I had never pressured her. " Over the following months their sexual contact was very enjoyable, fun and spontaneous, although the progression of their relationship was strikingly slow, at least according to Mrs. Carter. Eventually, she surprised him by saying she was on the pill and had had enough of waiting.

The first attempt at intercourse was painful and clumsy. Over the course of 20 years, their sex life had deteriorated gradually. At first, it was Mrs. Carter who initiated sex. Mrs. Carter said she loved having sex to make her husband happy. She had orgasms but no delight. Mr. Carter had never felt comfortable or been effective at making his wishes known. They both tended to follow all the rules they had somehow assimilated while growing up, including don't start anything you can't finish; any touch could lead to sex; sex should be all or nothing; sex must be natural and spontaneous; and talking ruins the mood.

Therapy Process

I requested a detailed description of "sex" and their feelings during sex. Their account is utterly dispassionate: Historically, about three-quarters of the time he says, "Let's go upstairs." She adds, "We go upstairs pretty well. I've never refused him. It's not an issue. The kids are asleep. It's at night. Then I'd change in the bathroom and put on a nightgown. He'd be in bed, waiting. I'd get in and we'd touch and kiss." For how long? She answers, "For 1 to 3 minutes. If I wasn't really in the mood, than it would be more like 1 minute. After 1 to

3 minutes, we would initiate intercourse. I still get sore when he first starts to penetrate ... but penetration is slow." "How slow is it?" I ask. They both agree: "About 10 seconds." Intercourse begins in the missionary position or with her on top for 2 minutes. Then he ejaculates. "Or if I try but it hurts too much when he starts to penetrate, I usually masturbate him." Mr. Carter adds, "Or I'll touch her breasts and make love with her breasts ... or she'll give me oral sex. I'll offer to give her oral sex and she'll say 'don't.' Then we talk for a minute or two and clean up. At one time it was exciting and I'd feel turned on. Not so much anymore." Mrs. Carter states, "Now it's less exciting but still loving because I know I'm making him happy ... but now there are more and more times where I feel nothing." Upon further inquiry, she adds, "I'm very uptight. I have a hard time relaxing and letting go. I need control. The only thing I can control is my body."

Fortunately the ideal they both aspire toward is similar: They seek sex that is "Fun, easygoing ... feeling close and together, so in love!" I agreed to help them replace dread with anticipation, but I could not assure them of what that sex might look like or what precisely they might come to anticipate. I did, however, note the absence of the erotic dimension in their description of their sex life and gave feedback accordingly, saying that I was not sure I'd want to have sex if I had their sex life, either. (It usually comes as a great relief to clients to hear this sentiment expressed.)

At the next session, Mrs. Carter commented that the initial meeting had been helpful. "We're talking more and differently ... We feel like a team." They seemed less blaming and accusatory. I asked Mrs. Carter to describe the best sex of her life. She recounted times in her late teens when she and Mr. Carter were dating. She recalled the stirrings she felt as the two sat in the backseat of his car, listening to the radio and "making out." These vague memories led us to look for moments of more intense arousal during those encounters. She recalls, "It made me feel really powerful that I turned him on." We identified a series of incidents in which she felt suffused with excitement and power at recognizing her capacity to arouse her boyfriend, to make him melt, and to turn him into the proverbial putty in her hands. These feelings were accompanied by a rush of heart-pounding energy, a sense of glee and delight at her own, long-forgotten ability to call the shots and make him want more—in fact, to make him want *her* more. As she lived in these moments, all of her senses were engaged. She particularly reveled in stroking him to the beat of the background music, switching her rhythm as dictated by the next song on the radio, and smelling him sweat with desire and anticipation during the lull between songs.

Homework in this approach typically originates from the client, who will try out new ways of being and behaving outside the office that had been recovered during the therapy session, Alternately, whatever homework assignments I might recommend—in contrast to those that come from the client—are always designed to elicit strong feeling.

The "homework" for the following session was dictated by the seductive young woman now sitting in my office toward the end of the session rather than by me, the therapist, or even by Mrs. Carter as she had been for most of her adult life. Mr. and Mrs. Carter were to take the car out to their favorite teen "make-out" spot, the woods alongside the Ottawa River Parkway, to put their compilation of 80s hits on the car stereo, and to play and explore sexually just as they had done in their teens.

At the next session, Mrs. Carter reported that they had aimed to "make out" for an hour. Mr. Carter said, "I enjoyed knowing there was no sex planned and only mutual exploration for its own sake." Mrs. Carter reported, "Yes, I get to *sensual* but not to *sexual*. An hour seems like forever ... All that's been on my mind is trying to fix this. What if I go through all of this and it still doesn't work in the end?" Clearly, Mrs. Carter had turned the homework she had designed herself into an evaluation of performance. "There's been no progress although our communication and interaction are better." Mr. Carter commented that her assessment of progress revealed a great deal about her definitions of sex and success. She complained that it was hard to know how to proceed. "I don't know what I like."

In the weeks that followed, Mr. and Mrs. Carter spent considerable time trying to discover what they liked. I told them to spend some time, perhaps 15 minutes each, *asking* for all the pleasure they could take and then attempt to actually receive it. This seems like a relatively simple bit of "homework" but it is deceptively difficult. For 20 years or so I have had clients experiment with this exercise, and it is a rare couple indeed who can stay with their feelings in their first effort for more than 15 minutes, as they encounter barriers within, interpersonally, and in the environment. The reports of their endeavors, of course, provide useful clinical material for developing embodiment, that is, the ability to be fully alive, present, and engaged in one's body (Kleinplatz & Ménard, 2007). It was quite illuminating for Mr. and Mrs. Carter. Their first attempt had brought home to them immediately the extent to which they aim to follow unspoken expectations rather than actually paying attention to what might prove pleasurable. Mrs. Carter had instructed him to do whatever *he* wanted, thereby revealing how she subverts her own attempts to discover what pleases her. As she put it, "Sex for me has been divided into, first I have 10 minutes of pleasure and then he has 10 minutes of sex." She added, "Touching him over the last weeks has been loving and sad. I felt badly that we had gotten so distant over the years. We had had a very 'TV image' of sex that said a woman needs touching and then a man needs an orgasm."

For Mr. Carter, "it was very sensual being touched." However, he was beginning to be confronted with his own inhibitions: "I'm reluctant to make myself vulnerable by having to ask ... for anything."

In the weeks that followed, Mr. and Mrs. Carter continued to experiment with asking for what gave them maximal pleasure, each time coming up against their own barriers to seeking out what they wanted most. These included fears of being selfish, being perceived as demanding or greedy, fears of being exposed, rejected, or losing control, and body image concerns. Over the course of the next four sessions we would work with whichever of these issues seemed to be most salient, evoking the most intense feelings during their explorations in bed and, especially, right then and there during the session.

At the outset of the fourth session, Mrs. Carter stated, "I don't believe him when he says he finds me extremely attractive. He's the perfect guy." Mr. Carter declared again his strong attraction for her. She discounted that, but more important her focus moved in another direction: "My worst fear is that he'd do the same thing as all the other people in my life and just leave, just like my dad." Her husband interrupts in a well-meaning attempt to offer reassurance. Nonetheless, she gives expression to her mounting fears of abandonment, of being seen as inadequate and left alone. "That's why it's so important to me to fulfill you sexually." Mr. Carter responded, "I've given you no indication ever that I'd ever leave." But she continued, becoming tearful, oblivious to his words, "No one has ever stuck around. I'm always afraid that I'll do one thing wrong and he'll leave."

I ask her to take me to the moments in her life when the fears she is now describing seemed most intense and threatening. We return to high school, which was replete with moments of rejection and abandonment. "I liked guys but it wasn't reciprocated, or not for long, because I wouldn't 'put out.' I liked this boy Jason for over a year. We finally went out and then he stopped talking to me. He had a huge crush on my best friend. I found out later he was going out with her, Beverly the perfect." As we explore these moments, speaking directly to the unavailable objects of her desire, we first come upon her pain, her feelings of being devastated and utterly crushed. Her chest is tight, heavy, and her heart is beating too fast. As we stay with these moments and delve deeper, something new begins to surface. We discover her unknown capacity to simply let go, to walk away unscathed, unharmed, to be separate, unique, distinct, and perhaps somewhat above her phalanx of false friends. Being apart from Jason—or her father—was beginning to feel like a relief. Staying with her husband suddenly felt like a choice made freely rather than an act of desperation to ward off the dread of being alone. As she turned to her husband, wondering what he had made of such intense self-revelation, he responded, "I'm not going anywhere. I *was never* going anywhere. I've been here for 20 years. When am I off probation? I don't want to go anywhere else and that's not going to change." Each of them relaxed, sighing audibly. As Mrs. Carter said, "That's good because I've decided you're a keeper. [Laughing] That helped quite a bit. The tightness is gone. I need to pay more attention to my body." They hugged just before they left the room.

Over the next month they continued to experiment with asking for all the pleasure they could take, but the exercise became more playful and the allotted time seemed to pass quickly so they increased their playtime. They began spending more time together and found different ways of being intimate, for example, going for walks, touching on the couch, and showering. In addition, they both noticed that they had forgone sexual intercourse but were spending a lot of time in mutual oral sex. The "rules" they had lived by began to disappear, especially the idea that sex and sexual arousal were all or nothing. As Mr. Carter said, "So it's not an 'on-or-off switch'— it's a dimmer."

In couples with sexual desire discrepancy, both initially tend to define one of them, (i.e., "the identified patient") as having low desire, as being defective and in need of fixing. Both tend to define the other partner as having a robust, healthy sexual appetite and as being ever ready, willing, and able to have sex if not for the obstacle of the reluctant partner. This ubiquitous pattern tends to maintain the status quo by keeping the couple polarized and each individual entrenched in a role that is really more of a caricature. For as long as these roles they have co-constructed remain unchallenged, neither one has to look too carefully at the purpose of the apparent "symptom"—it is much simpler to seek out the causes of psychopathology than to acknowledge the purpose of these polarized roles. When they begin to shift, there is often a sense of giddy disbelief and accompanying lightness and freedom that is quite palpable in the therapy room.

In this case, it was Mrs. Carter who had been constructed as the sole obstacle to sexual paradise. However, as soon as she began to change, it became increasingly obvious that Mr. Carter had been standing in his own way. His patiently waiting months for Mrs. Carter to be "ready" when they were still virgins was explained at the time as him having been a gentleman. His reluctance to initiate in the years that followed was attributed to his fear of being rebuffed by his beloved wife. It was only when she began to know what she wanted that it became apparent that Mr. Carter had been all too comfortable in the role of long-suffering and loyal husband who would never pressure his wife for sex. It was now time for him to take some chances, if he dared. Although this prospect initially seemed daunting to Mr. Carter, he quickly began to relish transcending his self-imposed boundaries and risking his own sexual self-expression.

One particularly important turning point occurred during one of Mr. Carter's turns to ask for pleasure. Mrs. Carter had been expecting instruction to give him manual or oral penile stimulation and was shocked when all he wanted was for her to caress his forearm. She kept preparing to reach for his penis and he would return her hand back to his forearm. He wanted a gentle, feathery touch, so light as to be barely discernible but just enough to make her presence known. As he later described it, "I finally got the idea that it was important to take responsibility for my own pleasure. I showed her what I wanted and it was a surprise ... " "To both of us!" She interjected. He continued, "I found it very arousing. I was trying different things but wanting her to touch me *just so* and *saying* so. I felt present and free. Afterward, she said she'd never felt closer to me." She added, "I felt warm, safe, loved, connected. I wanted to do this, even though it seemed a little weird until I got into it." Mr. Carter said, "Later, I felt at peace, calm ... really great. Nothing else mattered." Mrs. Carter commented, "Knowing that it's possible took the pressure off." Both finally felt they deserved whatever pleasure they wanted.

The fifth session marked the major turning point in therapy. In previous sessions, Mrs. Carter had mentioned her self-consciousness about her body without much feeling. In contrast, in the fifth session, as she begins to describe how she needs everyone to like the way she looks, "to have everyone accept me and like me, at my own expense," something more seems to be stirring. We begin the first step of this Experiential session: As I ask her to take us to a moment when these feelings seemed to be stronger, more pronounced, she describes her relationship with her friend Jennifer. "She was aggressive, closed-minded, and would cut you off. I organized their baby shower at her home and not one nice word from her. Only criticisms. I was shaking, I was so angry." At the time, Karen had been frozen and silent. The most palpable feeling at this point in the session is of her being passive in her habitual "people pleaser" mode that verges on martyrdom. She feels hurt, used, and unappreciated. However, during this session, we return to the baby shower and Karen confronts Jennifer, giving expression to her feelings at that time. She is saying, "I don't like the way you treat me. You don't do that if you have a real friendship. Everything always had to be the way you wanted. You are just miserable to be with. *Why did I ever care?*" As she says these words, something is beginning to emerge. She continues as the feelings intensify and peak: "I made huge changes in my life. Jennifer, I think you're jealous." The tight, frozen constricted feelings are dissolving: "I feel good. It's in my stomach. I'm feeling heard. What a relief! I used to think it was me." The heavy constricted feeling is gone and although it did not seem particularly difficult before, breathing now comes easier. There is a pleasant feeling of lightness and emptiness.

Here, in the key moment of the first step, we have found something in Mrs. Carter that is not normally accessible, but it is palpable and present in the course of the session. In the second step, Mrs. Carter takes a few more moments to identify and welcome this new potential. It is the sense of assertiveness, taking charge and entitlement accompanied by a freedom and expansiveness uncommon in her life.

During the third step of this session, we look for and locate other moments earlier in Mrs. Carter's life when such feelings occurred or should have occurred. We return to them with the intent to live in them fully and allow whatever was deeper within Mrs. Carter to surface. Mrs. Carter finds a whole series of painful events in her relationship with her mother. We enter into each one, looking for those most fraught with the newly available ways of being, whether or not they were accessible at the time. She recalls, "When I was a child, I was not allowed to snack. I was to eat what she served when she served it—never more and never less. One day in grade five I had a sleepover at a friend's house and we had blueberry pancakes for breakfast. When I got home I was nauseated but I was mostly afraid. Eventually, I had to tell her the truth because I knew I wasn't up to going to church. She never believed anything I said. She was going to send me anyhow until I started vomiting blueberries. She always lied so she assumed I did, too. I sat there on the bathroom floor, sick to my stomach while she yelled at me. I was such a mess." As we reenter this moment of cowering on the bathroom floor, she is emboldened even as she feels nauseated. This time, she literally stands up to her mother and starts hurling all over her mother's Sunday best. Little Karen Carter is feeling taller by the minute as she yells, "I've had enough of you. I'll eat what I want, when I want, where I want, and I'm not going to put up with your rules ever again. Do you hear me, Ethel? No, don't you dare hit me because you know I'll hit you back."

From there we are suddenly transported to grade 12 when Karen Carter was invited to visit Parliament Hill for fireworks on Canada Day. Karen was never permitted to have friends over but her home was the closest to the fireworks. When her friends dropped by to use the bathroom, "Mom came in. She slapped me in front of my friends *at the age of 17*! I was horrified. She actually smacked me in front of all those people, hard enough to leave hand prints. I spoke my mind. And then she did it again! She slapped me in the face for talking back! I learned early not to express my feelings. For the first time in my life, I thought I was actually going to hit her. I cannot believe that this is happening to me. This is what it's been like my whole life."

Only this time, as we go further in what might have been that day, Karen is looking at her mother and shouting back: "How can you do this to me, again?" They are right in each other's face. "You've never been a parent. I don't know what you are. You are a stupid, stupid woman. I don't think you really know how much damage you've done. I need my husband and friends to love me in the way you never did, and you still don't. I deserved better. I always did and I still do. You never cared about me. You should have *adored* me! Any other mother would have been *proud* to have me as her daughter … would have *treasured* me!" As she says these words, she is full of assertiveness and entitlement, but her voice has taken on a new tone, of feeling worthy, attractive, maybe even valuable. As if she is commenting to an imaginary audience, Mrs. Carter pronounces, "*I never felt entitled to the things I have. But not anymore!*"

During the fourth step, as Mrs. Carter begins to imagine how her life might be different if she treated herself as the special, valuable woman now unfolding in my office, a whole slew of possibilities bursts forth: "I could buy new clothes, get a gym membership, or go on more trips to the tropics. I could take a day and go to a spa for a massage, get a facial, a manicure, and get my hair all done pretty for no reason at all. Then I could get a nice dress and go out for dinner. I could go shopping for a really expensive pair of red high-heeled, open-toed pumps at the mall." She contemplated also writing a letter to her mother, "telling Mom what I felt all those years with an itemized invoice—I don't have to send it, but I might!" "I could go *crazy in bed … I could take charge, know what I want, pure pleasure and purely selfish*; I could stand up for myself at work with that arrogant boss and coworker Mary. I'm doing a hell of a standup job. Feels good to actually say it." Indeed she felt a loosening in her chest and stomach. Mrs. Carter continued triumphantly, "No more trying to please people who don't deserve to be pleased!"

Before leaving my office, Mrs. Carter committed to actually enacting at least two of the possibilities she had imagined, thereby making it more likely that the new person who had appeared during the session would continue to live and breathe in Mrs. Carter's "real" world. Mrs. Carter did, in fact, buy that pair of sexy new pumps later that day at the shoe boutique and did seek out pure pleasure in bed that night with a sense of joyous entitlement to sexual delight.

At our sixth session, Mr. and Mrs. Carter stated that they had made time alone together a priority and were having a lot of fun. "It was like being kids again. We've been playing strip poker." They had been exploring one another's bodies and had enjoyed touching and nibbling passionately. Mr. Carter commented, "It was so completely stress free, relaxed, and so connected." Mrs. Carter said, "I liked kissing his back … and cuddling later. It was me who initiated 'bringing it to the next level' with *no expectation or pressure*." They giggled as they searched for the words to describe their new pastime, " … Dry humping … It worked very well. We both had orgasms. It felt natural, intimate, in flow, in tune, in the moment … it felt right." Mr. Carter said, "I felt really connected and close to you." Mrs. Carter responded, "There was no pressure and no mental clouding. When we're there in that moment, that's where we're supposed to be. Just a complete focus on each other." And as Mr. Carter added, "There's no pressure as to how soon we'll do it again next."

Obviously, both were now enjoying their sex life and noted that although they were having sex more frequently, their idea of "progress" had been redefined. Mrs. Carter noted, "It's changed dramatically ... the new concept is of no expectation." Mr. Carter responded, "There are no more clouds ... instead we have a sense of optimism." Both were bubbling over with enthusiasm as Mrs. Carter said, "I feel much more desire than before. I'd like it to be higher still and that will come. I'm much more positive." They announced that they were ready to stop seeing me and agreed to a follow-up session 6 months later and another at the 18-month mark.

Therapy Outcome

Six months later, Mr. and Mrs. Carter were continuing to relate more and more openly and were touching more, both in and out of bed. Their frequent neck rubs in the living room had seemed so inviting that their youngest daughter had jumped in, wanting to participate. This in turn had led them to begin talking more openly with their children about sexuality, "sex education," and the role of sex in relationships. Reflecting back on her "progression" from youthful exploration to sexual intercourse, Mrs. Carter pointed out, "I realize now that once we began having 'sex' we cut back on pleasure." She wanted her children to have every option—not merely those prescribed by social norms.

They had arranged a weekend away and Mr. Carter had bought some lingerie that Mrs. Carter had worn for an evening out, building anticipation. "She looked hot!" Mr. Carter exclaimed and she responded, "Yeah, I really felt sexy there!" Mrs. Carter's body image and safety issues had now fully dissipated. She was now not only more comfortable in her own body but also more confident at work and with her mother. "I feel more often that I am likable, worth loving, and can be assertive without worrying." As they came to uncover each other more nakedly, they had begun to share fantasies and, in turn, as they ventured further, encountered more limits. For example, Mr. Carter noted, "I'm also coming up against my own inhibitions regarding initiation. I'm trying to seduce you, even though I prefer to be passive." One and one-half years later, the couple was continuing to blossom. They had entered a dialectical process in which each new discovery led to new erotic challenges to play with and overcome, if they so chose (Kleinplatz, 1992, 1996). Both reported focusing more fully, "no longer jumping ahead," "noticing more of what was going on," and "staying in the moment more." As Mr. Carter said in conclusion, "Our intimacy has become an oasis."

COMMENTARY

The outcome of this case was quite satisfying. It is characteristic of most of the cases I deal with in terms of the presenting problem, the histories of the couple, both as individuals and together, the nature, extent, and duration of their sexual desire discrepancy, the therapy provided, the goals achieved, and the couple's satisfaction with the results of therapy.

Two threads of interwoven factors contributed to the success of this case. The first is that the personal growth of these two individuals, particularly Mrs. Carter, allowed her to be more the kind of person she was meant to be. In Mrs. Carter's case, this entailed becoming more assertive and powerful, standing up for herself, and feeling valuable, worthy, and even desirable in her life in general and therefore in her sexuality as well. The nature of the sexual encounters shifted, because the people involved in them had changed in ways that were not specific to sex but encompassed sex. The second is that Mr. and Mrs. Carter redefined, expanded, and increased what they expected of sexuality. They stopped counting sexual events and began to engage in the kinds of sexual intimacy that were worthy of their efforts and were fulfilling.

Therapy allowed Mrs. Carter to access the experiencing within; to identify and welcome those ways of being; to live fully in the moments when that experiencing could have and should have surfaced; to be the person during the session she might have been all along; and to anticipate with glee the possibility of being this person in bed with Mr. Carter as well as in other contexts in the future. In addition, Mrs. Carter glimpsed how delightful it might be to actually live in this fashion during the sessions vividly enough so that she was enabled to carry this out in her everyday life. This led to changes in her relationship with her body and with Mr. Carter, (sexually and otherwise), as well as with other people, including her mother and her coworker. These changes, in turn, spurred Mr. Carter to see some opportunities for his own development, and the process looked so appealing that he, too, chose to grow.

Although it has been noted often in the literature that cases of low desire or sexual desire discrepancy are difficult to deal with effectively, that has not been my experience. Most of the men and women in my practice are seen for an average of 6 to 10 sessions. The changes occurring over the course of these sessions tend to be enduring, as seen at 18-month follow-up.

I wonder sometimes if the reason that cases of low desire are reported to be challenging is because the target of therapy a priori is increasing sexual frequency. First, to the extent that therapists are aiming to ameliorate a sexual *behavior*, in an area so central to identity and fraught with meaning, the resulting changes may be fleeting. However, the magnitude of change may be circumscribed by the limitations of the goals per se. On the other hand, when the goal of therapy is substantive personality change and presenting complaints are used as an entry point into the client's inner world, much broader, deeper, and enduring changes are possible (Mahrer, 1996). This case illustrates the value of an alternative approach: because Mrs. Carter made some fundamental changes in her personality, many things shifted; her sexuality and her sexual relations were only the icing on the cake.

Aside from the particular new ways of being unique to these individuals, a consequence of the therapy process is that the persons having the sex were more authentic, embodied, and alive and thus able to be more present, open, and free in their sexual and other relations. To the extent that therapy succeeds in helping individuals in relationships to fulfill their own potentials, should they choose to be sexual together that sex will become more optimal.

Second, this case illustrates the value of acknowledging the sorry state of the couple's sex life and the therapist's supporting them in refusing to settle for sexual drudgery. When individuals lose interest in sex, or at least in the caliber of sex they are currently rejecting, there is likely a *good reason*. Rather than helping patients to increase sexual frequency with minimal attention to the quality of their sexual relations, we might instead encourage clients *not* to have sex unless and until they know what they want, can ask for it, and feel flooded with erotic desire (Kleinplatz, 1992, 2006). One reason clients are reluctant to have "sex" is because they have an inkling from somewhere within or—for the lucky ones—some memories of what they really want.

I suppose one might argue that the changes in Mr. and Mrs. Carters sex life could be attributed to a change in their sexual script and therefore their sexual practices, allowing them to be more inclusive and to focus on sexual pleasure rather than sexual performance. I could appreciate this way of conceiving of the changes effected through therapy and would not quite argue with this characterization. However, this characterization does not address the more fundamental level at which change occurred. This couple did not replace their narrow and constricting notions of sex with others coming from the therapist; rather, because they changed as individuals and as a couple, new, more fulfilling options sprang from within and led to more optimal sexual intimacy. Although the majority of clients with low desire whom I see in therapy ultimately end up having more optimal sex, sex that is more authentic, uninhibited, erotically intimate, and intensely connected, the particulars remain unique to each individual or couple.

REFERENCES

Kleinplatz, P. J. (1992). The erotic experience and the intent to arouse. *Canadian Journal of Human Sexuality, 1*(3), 133–139.

Kleinplatz, P. J. (1996). The erotic encounter. *Journal of Humanistic Psychology, 36*(3), 105–123.

Kleinplatz, P. J. (1998). Sex therapy for vaginismus: A review, critique and humanistic alternative. *Journal of Humanistic Psychology, 38*(2), 51–81.

Kleinplatz, P. J. (1999). Infertility, "Experientially Oriented" couples therapy and subsequent pregnancy. *Journal of Couples Therapy, 8*(2), 17–35.

Kleinplatz, P. J. (2004). Beyond sexual mechanics and hydraulics: Humanizing the discourse surrounding erectile dysfunction. *Journal of Humanistic Psychology, 44*(2), 215–242.

Kleinplatz, P. J. (2006). Learning from extraordinary lovers: Lessons from the edge. *Journal of Homosexuality, 50*(3/4), 325–348.

Kleinplatz, P. J. (2007). Coming out of the sex therapy closet: Using experiential psychotherapy with sexual problems and concerns. *American Journal of Psychotherapy, 61*(3), 333–348.

Kleinplatz, P. J., & Krippner, S. (2005). Spirituality and sexuality: Celebrating erotic transcendence and spiritual embodiment. In S. G. Mijares & G. S. Khalsa (Eds.), *The psychospiritual clinician's handbook: Alternative methods for understanding and treating mental disorders* (pp. 301–318). Binghamton, NY: Haworth.

Kleinplatz, P. J., & Ménard, A. D. (2007). Building blocks towards optimal sexuality: Constructing a conceptual model. *The Family Journal: Counseling and Therapy for Couples and Families, 15*(1), 72–78.

Kleinplatz, P. J., Ménard, A. D., Paquet, M.-P., Paradís, N., Campbell, M. Zuccarini, D., & Mehak, L. (2009). The components of optimal sexuality: A portrait of "great sex." *Canadian Journal of Human Sexuality, 18*(1-2), 1–13.

Mahrer, A. R. (1978). *Experiencing: A humanistic theory of psychology and psychiatry.* New York: Brunner/Mazel.

Mahrer, A. R. (1996). *The complete guide to Experiential Psychotherapy.* Boulder, CO: Bull Publishing.

Mahrer, A. R. (2002). *Becoming the person you can become: The complete guide to self-transformation.* Boulder, CO: Bull Publishing.

Mahrer, A. R. (2008a). *The manual of optimal behaviors.* Montreal: Howard Gontovnick.

Mahrer, A. R. (2008b). *The optimal person.* Montreal: Howard Gontovnick.

Mahrer, A. R., & Boulet, D. B. (2001). How can Experiential Psychotherapy help transform the field of sex therapy? In P. J. Kleinplatz (Ed.), *New directions in sex therapy: Innovations and alternatives* (pp. 234–257). Philadelphia: Brunner-Routledge.

Chapter 7

A Skeptical View of Desire Norms and Disorders Promotes Clinical Success

Leonore Tiefer
Marny Hall

In this chapter, Leonore Tiefer and Marny Hall illustrate the possibilities of treating sexual desire complaints from a nonpathological model. Rather than using the DSM-IV-TR criteria as a tool for diagnosing sexual desire problems, they rely on the New View classification, which considers sexual complaints within a cultural context and serves as a guide for assessment and treatment.

Because these authors regard sexual desire as culturally determined and socially scripted, they avoid using the language of "sex drive." They believe that this term reinforces the mistaken belief that sexual desire is intrinsic, internal, and biologically based. Rather they see sex as a learned, scripted, and socially "normed" behavior. They suggest that a sex therapist can function as a coach who facilitates sensual, recreational, emotional, and attitudinal learning and growth. In fact, they assert that an ethical therapist should refrain from allying with cultural norms regarding sexuality but rather help couples sort out the kind of sensual and romantic life that works best for them, even if it completely omits traditional "coupling." Finally, they avoid endorsing any one path to clinical success, believing that each case must be assessed and treated uniquely without preconceived goals or interventions.

These authors illustrate the various ways in which the New View classification may guide treatment by presenting three short cases, one involving a lesbian couple, another a traditional heterosexual couple, and the third a couple struggling with personality and recreational differences. The three cases have different outcomes, and actual changes in sexual frequency are modest or absent altogether. Nevertheless, it would be difficult to argue that these are not successful outcomes. Instead of linking assessments of success (or failure) solely to sexual performance and frequency, the New View—by naming and challenging conventional standards of sexual success and failure—invites clinicians to use richer and more nuanced ways of assessing outcome in sex therapy.

Leonore Tiefer, PhD, is Clinical Associate Professor (Psychiatry) at New York University School of Medicine. She is the author, among other works, of *Sex Is Not a Natural Act* (2nd ed.) and founded the Campaign for a New View of Women's Sexual Problems (*newviewcampaign.org*) in 2000.

Marny Hall, PhD, LCSW, is a sex therapist in the San Francisco Bay area. Her books include *The Lavender Couch, Sexualities, The Lesbian Love Companion,* and, with Kimeron Hardin, *Queer Blues.*

INTRODUCTION: THERE CAN BE NO VALID DIAGNOSTIC SCHEME, BUT THERE CAN BE USEFUL CLASSIFICATION SYSTEMS

There have been rules and recommendations regarding sexual desire and sexual activity throughout recorded history (Nye, 1999). Some proclaim the dangers of indulgence, some the perils of restraint. Depending on the author and his or her occupation and cultural background, standards have been more or less based on gender and race, written in Latin or the vernacular, promoted from pulpits or through broadsides.

Twentieth-century Western science entered the arena of sexual norms in the form of official postwar medical classification schemes such as that proposed by the American Psychiatric Association in 1952 and repeatedly revised thereafter (American Psychiatric Association, 1994). At first largely ignored outside psychiatry, sexual function nomenclature has drawn increasing attention in the past decade in research and at conferences supported by a new global industry devoted to medical function treatment.

A plethora of new science-focused sexuality texts use the language of health and the rhetoric of "evidence-based" to draw lines between acceptable and problematic forms of sexual desire and expression. Despite the technical jargon, however, there is no more consensus on how much or little interest in sex is normal or healthy than there was in "prescientific" eras on how much or little sexual interest was chaste, undisciplined, pious, or dishonorable.

We believe that there can *never* be a successful way to define good/normal/healthy/correct sexual desire outside of cultural standards for the simple reason that sexual desire is a product of human psychobiological development and expression permanently controlled, contained, and constructed by cultural context. Current official scientific formulations draw on a mythical universal model of sexual response, locating the desire for sexual expression in an alleged and romanticized model of species-specific and species-wide biological/hormonal/genetic origins. But any examination of the innumerable permutations of sexual meaning, social priority, and expressive form, especially one grounded in a knowledge of the history of human sexuality, pulls the rug out from under this mythical "human sexual response."

PEOPLE LOOK FOR GUIDELINES AND MEDIA INFLATE INSECURITY

Nevertheless, although there can be no objective or universal answer to the question of what type or amount of sexual expression is normal, the "proper" performance of sexual activity is highly valued in many cultures as a sign of individual maturity and gender adequacy. Satisfaction with sex is widely viewed as an indispensible element in relationship success and longevity. Mass media, most people's source of sexuality education, endlessly celebrates proper sexual performance in print, film, and on the Web. Knowing and conforming to age- and gender-appropriate standards is of widespread interest and personal concern. Although many websites now inclusively advise that "everybody's different and everybody's normal when it comes to sex and sexuality" (e.g., *sexualityandu.ca*, 2008) and magazines advertise "helpful tips" from their colorful covers, paradoxically the attention to sexual performance, even when it is supposed to reassure, often generates and escalates insecurity.

THE NEW VIEW APPROACH
AND CLASSIFICATION SCHEME

Noticing the increasing public attention to sexual norms and concerned that medical professionals and an ambitious pharmaceutical industry were promoting false standards and exploiting the public's insecurities, a group of feminist social scientists and health professionals met in 2000 to analyze the situation and develop an approach to classification that could be used to guide sex education and treatment *without imposing norms.* The resulting New View manifesto has been widely published and its classification system has been presented in workshops and educational venues (Working Group for a New View of Women's Sexual Problems, 2000; *newviewcampaign. org*) (Table 7.1). Originally developed to apply to women, the system was reworked slightly in 2006 to be useful for educating and treating men as well (Tiefer, 2006).

One of the two crucial elements of the New View approach is its definition of sexual problems. The classification guidelines state (see Table 7.1), "Sexual problems are *defined* by the Working Group as discontent or dissatisfaction with *any* emotional, physical, or relational aspect of sexual experience" (emphasis added). The New View approach allows people to define their own problems, assuming, in the absence of universal norms, that discontent or dissatisfaction is a matter of wide individual and couple variation. This is to be contrasted with the definition in the American Psychiatric Association's manual that specifies sexual problems as disturbances in hypothesized norms, that is, "the [*sic*] sexual response cycle." "The sexual dysfunctions are characterized by disturbance in sexual desire and in the psychophysiological changes that characterize the sexual response cycle and cause marked distress and interpersonal difficulty" (American Psychiatric Association, 1994, p. 493).

For the clinician using the New View approach, the absence of norms for sexual desire offers some important therapeutic advantages:

- A secure position from which to construe differences in sexual interest between sexual partners as discrepancies *like other* relational discrepancies (e.g., whether to spend holidays with one set of in-laws or the other; whether to have children now, later, or not at all).
- A starting point for analysis and behavioral modification that

TABLE 7.1. The New View Classification System

Sexual problems are *defined* by the Working Group as discontent or dissatisfaction with *any* emotional, physical, or relational aspect of sexual experience. They may arise in one or more of the following four interrelated dimensions of people's sexual lives.

I. Sexual problems due to sociocultural, political, or economic factors
    A. Ignorance or anxiety due to inadequate sex education, lack of access to health services, or other social constraints including:
        1. Lack of vocabulary to describe subjective or physical experience.
        2. Lack of information about human sexual biology and life-stage changes.
        3. Lack of information about how gender roles and cultural norms influence men's and women's sexual expectations, beliefs, and behaviors.
        4. Inadequate access to information and services for contraception and abortion, STD prevention and treatment, sexual trauma, and domestic violence.

    B. Sexual avoidance, distress, or lack of pleasure due to perceived inability to meet cultural norms regarding correct or ideal sexuality, including:
        1. Anxiety or shame about one's body, sexual attractiveness, or sexual responses.
        2. Confusion or shame about one's sexual orientation or identity, or about sexual fantasies, desires, and preferences.
        3. Fear of judgment or punishment by cultural, community, or religious institutions.

    C. Inhibitions due to conflict between the sexual norms of one's subculture or culture of origin and those of the dominant culture.

    D. Lack of interest, fatigue, or lack of time due to family, work, or other obligations.

II. Sexual problems due to partner and relationship factors
    A. Inhibition, avoidance, or distress arising from:
        1. Betrayal, dislike, fear, or resentment of partner, abuse or exploitation by partner, or partners' unequal power status.
        2. Discrepancies in desire for frequency or nature of sexual activity.
        3   Inability to communicate effectively about preferences for initiation, pacing, or shaping of sexual activities.
        4. Disagreements, spoken or assumed, about the terms of the relationship, the degree or meaning of commitment, or the desire for monogamy or non-monogamy.

    B. Loss of sexual interest and reciprocity as a result of ongoing conflicts over commonplace issues such as money, schedules, or relatives, or resulting from traumatic experiences, such as infertility or the death of a child.

    C. Inhibitions in arousal or spontaneity in response to partner's health status or sexual problems.

III. Sexual problems due to psychological factors
    A. Experienced or perceived lack of choice in sexual behaviors or attitudes, ranging from aversion toward or ambivalence about sexual pleasure to sexual obsessions or compulsive behaviors.

    B. Consequences of past negative sexual, physical, or emotional experiences.

TABLE 7.1. (*continued*)

   C. Guilt or shame about sexual desires or fantasies.

   D. Effects of depression or anxiety.

   E. General personality problems with attachment, rejection, cooperation, or entitlement.

   F. Sexual inhibition due to possible negative consequences (e.g., pain during sex, pregnancy, sexually transmitted disease, loss of reputation, rejection, or abandonment by partner).

   G. Deeply held negative beliefs about one's self-worth or desirability.

   H. Not accepting age-related life changes.

IV. Sexual problems due to physiological or medical factors
Pain or lack of physical sensation or response during sexual activity despite a supportive and safe interpersonal situation, adequate sexual knowledge, and positive sexual attitudes. Such problems may arise from:

   A. Local or systemic medical conditions affecting neurological, vascular, circulatory, endocrine, musculoskeletal, or other systems of the body.

   B. Pregnancy, fertility treatments, sexually transmitted diseases, or other sex or reproductive conditions.

   C. Side effects of drugs, medications, or medical treatments.

   D. Overuse or dependence on alcohol or other recreational or prescribed drugs or other substances.

Note. Based on Tiefer (2006); unified language for both men and women.

minimizes partners' name-calling and interrupts efforts to ally with the "sexually normal" therapist.
- An immediate focus on cultural influences that can be used throughout treatment.
- An immediate focus on sexual habits and preferences as learned that can be used throughout treatment.

The other crucial element of the New View approach is its extensive listing of factors contributing to sexual distress and dissatisfaction, grouped into four categories (see Table 7.1):

- Sexual problems due to sociocultural, political, or economic factors
- Sexual problems due to partner and relationship factors
- Sexual problems due to psychological factors
- Sexual problems due to physiological or medical factors

The expansive lists of elements within each category draw the therapist's attention to the assorted and multifarious ways that cultural factors can contribute to sexual problems, offering opportunities for bibliotherapy, directions for focused sexual history taking, and ideas for clinical interventions and homework assignments.

In order to demonstrate how the New View approach guides the treatment of couples presenting with complaints involving sexual desire, three illustrative cases are presented. All were seen and treated by Marny Hall.

CASE EXAMPLE 1: KENJI AND MARSHA— POST-HONEYMOON BLUES

Kenji grew up in Taiwan. After her announcement that she was a lesbian created a hornet's nest of family protest, she fled to Northern California. Just 21 when she arrived in San Francisco, Kenji got a job as a taxi driver and plunged wholeheartedly into the gay scene. It was exhilarating to be free of family obligations and constraints. The oldest of three sisters, Kenji had—for as long as she could remember—felt responsible for her family's well-being. Her mother—ill and depressed—stayed in her bedroom for days at a time. Her father rarely came home. When Kenji was 10, she found out that his "business trips" had simply been weeklong gambling binges. By contrast, her new "chosen" San Francisco family of queer playmates was always supportive and available. Her new friends and lovers were also, for the most part, heavy drinkers and recreational drug users. It wasn't uncommon for Kenji to party all night with them and then segue, without any break, into her day shift at the cab company. When she was 25, she was pulled over for erratic driving. Her blood alcohol level was well over the legal limit. She lost her job and her driver's license and faced a stiff fine that the judge promised to waive on the condition that Kenji started going to AA. Kenji complied.

By the time she was 30, Kenji had been a regular AA member for 5 years, gotten an administrative job in an international banking firm, and hooked up with Marsha, another AA member. Like Kenji's relatives, Marsha's Polish Catholic family in Chicago raised a furor when she came out. She, too, left her home precipitously and headed for the gay-friendly Bay Area. New teaching credential in hand, she had no trouble landing a job as a math teacher in an inner city public school. Before she joined AA, Marsha had also burned the candle at both ends, working all day and partying hard at night. For her too this had been a welcome emancipation from family-of-origin travails. Marsha's father had been an alcoholic unable to keep a job. His premature death when Marsha was a teen left the family's fortunes even more precarious. Marsha's mother had to shuttle between two jobs to keep the family intact. Preoccupied with survival issues, she had little time or energy for Marsha or her four siblings. But, Marsha reported, the kids pulled together and nurtured each other in myriad ways. After they had recovered from the coming-out rupture, Marsha's family members were once again very close.

When they came for sex therapy, Kenji and Marsha were in their mid-30s and had been together for 6 years. They reported that, aside from their sexual impasse, they got along well together. They rarely disagreed and when they did have a conflict, they resolved the dispute easily. Marsha's gift for dissolving tension was apparent early in therapy. In the first session, they disagreed—somewhat heatedly—about who had made the first move toward a romantic connection. "Yes," Marsha said slyly, "you first asked me out for coffee but I had been vibing you for months before that—slinging it like this." Marsha then demonstrated her wiles by puckering her lips and batting her lashes at Kenji. At this, Kenji giggled and shrugged. The argument was over. When I commented on her conciliation talents, Marsha said that, as the middle child in a family of five, it had been her role to make peace between the older and younger kids.

Presenting Problem and History

During the initial session, Marsha and Kenji reported that their strenuous efforts to avoid "lesbian bed death" (LBD) had failed. Neither had any desire for sex. In their previous relationships with other partners, such a dramatic cessation of desire had presaged the end of the partnerships, and they were afraid that history would repeat itself and that they would lose each other.

The specter of LBD had haunted their relationship from its inception. It was legendary in their AA community. "U-haul lesbians"—those who moved in together on the second date—were reputed to be the most susceptible to LBD. According to conventional wisdom, becoming domesticated too quickly was a sure way to kill romance. In order to avoid such a fate, Kenji and Marsha had proceeded cautiously—stretching out their courtship for months. They were very attracted to one another and reported that lovemaking, when it finally happened, exceeded all expectations. They were "on cloud nine" for days afterward. Compelling as the sex was, they continued to pace their relationship in a deliberate way. Their determination to manage their relationship carefully, as well as their demanding commitments to work and to their AA programs, kept them apart during the week. As a consequence, weekends became much anticipated and treasured romantic interludes. After 2 years of sustained sexual passion for one another—certain that they had eluded the dreaded LBD—they moved in together.

They reported that over the next 2 years their desire faded imperceptibly. Intervals between lovemaking gradually increased from a few days to a week, to a month. Each reported keeping a secret tally of "how long it had been." To acknowledge any lapse in desire for one another would have confirmed that their efforts to avoid the dreaded LBD had failed, so they made excuses: they were too tired or too stressed about work or too avid about a new queer TV series to make time for lovemaking.

When San Francisco mayor Gavin Newsom legalized gay marriage in 2004, Kenji and Marsha planned their nuptials. They would go to City Hall, get married, then go to a friend's cabin for a weekend honeymoon. Discussion of the honeymoon plan finally broke their conspiracy of silence. They joked awkwardly about it. What if, once they got to the cabin, they didn't feel like sex? What kind of honeymoon would it be? It was after this mutual acknowledgment that they decided to pursue sex therapy.

Case Conceptualization and Treatment

A sex therapist applying American Psychiatric Association criteria to this situation of persistently deficient sexual desire might diagnose Kenji and Marsha as each suffering from hypoactive sexual desire disorder (HSDD). After arriving at such a diagnosis, a conventional sex therapist might prescribe a series of non-goal-oriented sensuality exercises as homework. According to conventional precepts, such a regimen would help the couple move toward resuming their previous erotic intimacy or at least reveal blocks to that intimacy.

In contrast, a New View–oriented practitioner would approach the problem from another angle, viewing Marsha and Kenji's sexual avoidance as based on shame stemming from "perceived inability to meet cultural norms regarding correct or ideal sexuality" (Table

7.1, I.B). Romance, desire, and passion are not simply the preferred narratives of the heterosexual culture. Before recent legal moves to legitimize gay relationships, passionate desire had been the sole criterion for validating lesbian relationships. Without the requisite erotic credentials, intimate relationships between women become invisible; cohabiting and committed partners are likely to be perceived as "just roommates." In the case of Marsha and Kenji, there is another twist to the "just roommate" narrative. Growing up, each partner was most validated in her role as sister, as it was Kenji's and Marsha's siblings—as opposed to parents or other relatives—who had provided each with affirmation and love. Therefore, for Kenji and Marsha, the role of sibling—with its associations of comfort, collaboration, and, not least important, its prohibition of sexuality—had provided the template for positive relationships.

Simply by virtue of being an authority figure who responds positively to the couple's history, the sex therapist is positioned to counter the shame and the sense of relationship inadequacy so often shared by partners. I expressed genuine awe about their success at making their passion last as long as it had. In fact, if anything, their campaign had perhaps been too successful. Because they had managed to sustain their erotic intensity for so long, Kenji and Marsha had inadvertently fused passion and sex. As a result other, less earth-moving inclinations toward intimacy, too subtle to register on their passion radar, probably escaped their notice. In other words, because sex between them had been so memorable, the only conditions salient enough to catch their attention were passionate desire or its polar opposite—LBD.

However, early in the therapy I observed that the couple's easy, low-key intimacy indicated that they often inhabited a middle ground between passion and LBD. I asked if they would be willing to pay more attention to this middle ground and proposed that we begin to look for ways to translate their playful qualities, their humor and irreverence, and their ease with each other into special forms of eroticism to challenge their narrow sexual paradigm. They were willing but dubious. They said they had come to therapy hoping to rekindle their honeymoon passion.

This was perhaps *the* critical point in therapy—a moment when I took a strong stand that diverged from cultural norms about sex and sex therapy. As directed by the New View approach, I explicitly challenged the prevailing essentialist model and norms of sex. I responded that, experienced as I was, I had never been able to help long-term couples re-create the circumstances that had once generated intense desire. For most couples, I had observed that passion sprang from some combination of novelty, uncertainty, and taboo-breaking—a constellation of elements that, if relationships endured, was unsustainable. Perhaps the most central aspect of our therapy, I said, would be expressing sadness about the transience of such ardor. Nevertheless, I added, even if passionate love was transitory, it nonetheless deserved their continuing homage. If they had never experienced intense desire for other women, they would never have become lesbians—a hard-won identity each woman valued. Most important, they never would have gotten together.

As their first homework assignment, I asked them to spend time together contemplating the shared erotic passion that each declared had been the most profound experience of her life. I proposed that they find a special candle—selected for its pleasing size, shape, and scent—and that they light it for 20 minutes every night for a week. During this ritual, I asked them to sit together and meditate quietly on Eros with their minds and hearts or whatever sensing and feeling faculties they could muster. If Aphrodite were thus honored, I observed (only half jokingly), she would help Kenji and Marsha make the necessary passage to other sorts of sensuality and pleasure. The point of this assignment was to counter the shame that Marsha and Kenji felt about the cessation of passionate desire in their relationship. The staging of such a ritual announces to the participants that—far from being over—this chapter in their lives, now enshrined, will continue to exist in a transcendent way. In the following session, they reported both grief and relief. They were, they said, receptive to the "middle ground" sex that I had proposed.

For their next homework assignment, I asked them to continue the candle-burning ritual. I also gave them two handouts to take home and discuss: a list of different sorts of love catalogued by the Greeks (Hall, 1998, p. 84), and Annie Sprinkle's *101 Uses for Sex— or Why Sex Is So Important* (Sprinkle, 1996, pp. 5–6). Among the various purposes Sprinkle lists are: "Sex as a sedative ... Sex as a reward ... Sex to make you laugh (it can be hilarious)." In the following session, we brainstormed still more counternormative variations such as maybe-I'll-feel-like-it-after-we-start sex, let's-just-do-you sex, no-big-deal quickies, if-I-don't-have-to-lift-a-finger sex, orgasm-free sex, and so on.

I asked them to experiment with their own alternative forms of intimacy. In the next session, Marsha reported piggybacking on a titillating childhood memory. As a 10-year-old, she had gotten "exams" from a school pal who had had a toy medical kit. After she reminisced with Kenji, they went to a secondhand medical supply store, got a nurse's uniform and some other supplies, and played "naughty nursey." This blend of friction and fantasy was a poor substitute for previous passion, they said, but it had been silly and fun. They were relieved to break the long dry spell. In the next sessions, we continued to discuss the loss of their desire and to come up with homework experiences that developed and reinforced the emerging paradigm.

A few weeks into therapy, following an Easter vacation trip home to Chicago, Marsha and Kenji reported that Marsha's mother's health was failing. During a family conference, Marsha had decided she had to move to Chicago to help, and Kenji agreed to the move as her company had available openings in Chicago. Marsha would have no trouble getting a teaching job. They planned to leave after the school year was over.

Therapy Tune-Ups

Kenji and Marsha terminated therapy and moved to Chicago 3 years ago. Because of continuing connections to the Bay Area, however, they make regular pilgrimages back to San Francisco, and whenever they return, they contact me for a "tune-up." Typically they report that their erotic momentum persists for a few months following each appointment with me. They do get turned on by the friction-and-fantasy formats they have developed, but at a certain point such postpassionate intimacies begin to feel contrived—too different from the effortless sex they experienced in their initial years together to be worth the exertion. I comment that their self-consciousness is a valid and valuable signal; it means that they are swimming against the cultural current of standardized sex norms that they, like the rest of us, have internalized as the "truth" of sex. I reemphasize the ubiquitous presence—in both queer and straight culture—of one-size-fits-all messages about sex. In the face of such powerful and pervasive influences, I observe, it is remarkable that they can invent and follow their own erotic scripts for even 10 seconds. By the end of these tune-up sessions, Kenji and Marsha are again eager to experiment with their own brand of intimacy. Each time they come back to see me, their own signature eroticism seems easier and more satisfactory. Both women are now almost 40, and have been together for almost a decade. Sex therapy continues to be, perhaps, a two-steps-forward, one-step-back process.

CASE EXAMPLE 2: ALAN AND GRACE—
THE CONSOLATIONS OF TOUCH

Presenting Problem and History

In their mid-30s, Alan and Grace are transplanted midwesterners from big farm families. They met at the Silicon Valley company where they work as software engineers. Both claimed their fall into love was a plunge, precipitous and thrilling. They married 6 months later. In the beginning, sex was superb—fueled by mutual passion and biological urgency. They wanted to start a family. As months, then years, ticked by and Grace did not get pregnant, they began to feel pressured. Following the regimen recommended by a fertility specialist, they tracked ovulation. Sex turned into a chore for Grace—a duty to be performed at appointed times. Still she did not get pregnant. They embarked on a series of expensive and invasive fertilization-enhancing procedures. After several setbacks (including two late miscarriages), Grace became pregnant again. Confined to bed for the second half of her pregnancy and outfitted with a monitor that would tell her if the baby's heart stopped, she successfully carried the baby to term. Without a moment to recover from months of stress and uncertainty, Alan and Grace became new parents ... and sexless partners. Alan was interested in sex, but no trace of Grace's early passion survived the protracted and painful attempts to have a child.

By the time they came to sex therapy, their son, Jordan, was an amiable and much-loved preschooler. Again, using the DSM criteria of persistently deficient sexual desire and the fact that Alan was unhappy with the sexless status quo, a sex therapist might diagnose HSDD (American Psychiatric Association, 1994). Applying traditional sex therapy, the clinician again might reasonably suggest that Alan and Grace begin a series of non-goal-oriented massages—exercises designed to rekindle Grace's presumably dormant desire.

Treatment and Discussion

Rather than assuming that an absence of sexual desire in and of itself is a problem, in this case the New View would finger relational trauma (i.e., "Loss of sexual interest and reciprocity as a result of conflicts ... resulting from traumatic experiences, e.g., infertility or the death of a child"; see Table 7.1. Section II, B) as the clinical issue. Acknowledging grief and stress (the specific vigilance occasioned by the miscarriages) was the starting point for sex therapy with this couple.

Grace continued to feel that Jordan's existence hung in the balance and, consequently, she monitored him closely. During an initial session, it was easy to expand this preexisting framework (preoccupation with the well-being of Jordan) with a piece of conventional wisdom: a robust relationship between Jordan's parents would provide the most nurturing possible environment for him. To achieve this, Alan and Grace needed time alone together to recover from the previous years' ordeal. Their psychological wounds deserved tending. Carving out time for healing interludes required our going over the details of child care. Nuts-and-bolts planning about reliable babysitters—though far removed from anything remotely erotic—was the key part of the couple's "sex" therapy. With a couple of hours cordoned off, they were instructed to simply spend soothing time together—relaxing, napping, spooning, having in-house picnics, reading together, or pursuing any other intimate activity they chose. After 2 weeks, they added shared showers and massages to their rest and recreation routines. Without any prompting, their interludes became erotic in new, calm, and tender ways.

During therapy, Grace and Alan discussed their surprising tentativeness with each other. They reminisced about their honeymoon period, as well as the sexual adventures—both positive and negative—that predated their relationship. Because they had a wide repertoire of experiences it was easy to segue to a discussion of cultural myths and messages about one-size-fits-all sex. After 2 months of weekly therapy, Alan and Grace left for a long-scheduled 3-week family vacation. They spent time with Alan's extended family at a mountain retreat. When they returned, they reported that thanks to relatives who were enthusiastic babysitters they were able to continue their time-outs. Sex, minus the old bells and whistles, had become a consolation, one way among many of being close and comforting each other.

CASE EXAMPLE 3: SEAN AND EVA— WIZARDS OF INTIMACY

Sean, 48, is an energy-saving consultant for large corporations, an antiwar activist, and a transplant from Ireland. He grew up in an emotionally arid household, as the middle of five sons in a Dublin slum. Despite his liberal politics, he described himself as sexually conservative. He had had few lovers and liked sex with the lights out, missionary style. Eva, the only daughter of Jewish union organizers, grew up in New York City, came to college in Berkeley in the 1980s, and never left. The director of a nonprofit company that provides services for newly arriving Latina immigrants, Eva had had many lovers—both casual encounters and live-in partners.

History

Sean and Eva were housemates before becoming lovers. They lived in a sprawling Victorian house with a group of like-minded activists. Over time, they began going to concerts and films together. When they realized they were attracted to each other, they moved out and found their own place. At first, sex was equally exciting for both. But over the next year, a misalignment emerged. Sean felt they didn't physically fit in a way that provided enough friction for him to maintain an erection or achieve orgasm and he lost interest in sex. After a long spell of frustration, followed by a stretch of complete abstinence, Eva insisted they see a sex therapist recommended by a friend. The therapist enlisted them in a slow-paced program of sensual massage and mutual masturbation. The goal of these at-home assignments was to become more familiar with one another's bodies, preferences, and pleasures. Eva hoped that Sean would become comfortable substituting the pleasures of "outercourse" for his preferred but nonworking intercourse.

Given the standard DSM approach that would label this a case of lost desire as a consequence of erectile disorder, such techniques seemed appropriate. Though Sean and Eva found the therapist helpful and sensitive, the exercises simply exacerbated their differences. They became polarized, Sean claiming he was just an old-fashioned guy and Eva losing her previous self-assurance. The whole area of sexuality became aversive. They stopped sex therapy and all attempts to have any kind of sex. A clinician might now diagnose the problem as a sexual aversion disorder. At Eva's urging, they agreed to see a new sex therapist.

Intervention

During their first visit both complained that after 7 years of living together, their misalignment persisted. They were as sexually incompatible as they were socially in sync. As a result of their prodigious efforts to cure the problem, sex had become an ordeal that they both avoided. Using the New View to classify the couple's avoidance not as a sexual disorder but as a partner issue of discrepant attitudes (specifically, a discrepancy regarding frequency or nature of sexual activity; see Table 7.1, II.A.2) removes any implication that the impasse is pathological and must, therefore, be cured or dissolved. Rather, such an analysis opens up the possibility of discussing that a couple's approach to sex, as to other hobbies and shared activities, exists on a continuum of compatibility. This discussion explicitly takes the pressure off partners to conform to a one-size-fits-all sexual intimacy.

In therapy, Sean and Eva were encouraged to explore what their erotic alignment and misalignment meant to each. Such a starting point stressed diversity rather than some "universal" sexual boilerplate. As the discussion proceeded, very diverse attitudes about the role of sex emerged. For Eva, who defined herself as "a very sexual person," sex was the sine qua non of partnership. For Sean, sex was a "take it or leave it" matter. He rarely masturbated and had been contentedly celibate for months at a time. As a young man, he had seriously considered the priesthood.

Once it was permissible to discuss, rather than fear, different views on sex, not surprisingly other differences could be acknowledged. Sean wanted to join the Peace Corps and live overseas; Eva was invested in her California job. He loved backpacking; she liked bicycling. As they had grown older, he had become more solitary, she more gregarious. It emerged that earlier in their relationship any mention of such differences had been taboo because of the worst-case scenario each privately dreaded: if they were incompatible as lovers, they would have to break up, acrimoniously and irrevocably. These beliefs, explored in therapy, had a variety of sources: bruising breakups each had experienced in the past; messages from both Eva's and Sean's parents that couples stick together through thick and thin; and perhaps most important, the ubiquitous happily-ever-after stories favored by popular culture.

Rather than their sexual functioning, the New View taxonomy pinpointed Sean and Eva's shame about not living up to norms as the area of clinical intervention. Together we considered the absence of familial or cultural support for any sort of bond that wasn't sexual. To fill in the cultural lacuna, we gave ourselves an assignment. I would try to find some written accounts of non-erotic but loving cross-sex bonds. Because they were film buffs, they promised to find films that featured loving nonsexual bonds between cross-sexed peers. When we met again, I reported that I was only able to find one book (Brain, 1976) and one magazine article (Chatterjee, 2001). They reported, laughing, that they too had been struck by how rarely such loving bonds are considered worthy of cinematic representation. They had only been able to find one film on the subject: *The Wizard of Oz*.

With their shame somewhat reduced, Sean and Eva were able to consider the pros and cons of continuing their live-in relationship. After long deliberation—much of it painful—they concluded they were superb friends and decided to move apart. Wrenching as this separation was, they negotiated it in a nonblaming, mutually supportive way. Six months after they stopped therapy, I bumped into Sean and Eva in a movie queue in Berkeley. Amused, they told me I'd caught them in flagrante delicto during one of their weekly film dates. They continue to be intimate in other ways. Sean has just nursed Eva through a nasty bout of flu. Eva tells me that she is interviewing candidates from an online dating service she has joined. Sean remains contentedly celibate.

Discussion

If we use the resumption of an erotic connection as the sole measure of therapeutic success, this case is a therapy failure. Not only was the therapist unable to facilitate a rekindling of desire in the partners; they ultimately separated. However, positive outcomes—using the New View approach—are measured within a broader context of client well-being. In the case of Sean and Eva, shame associated with their discrepancy in desire had been reinforced by the interventions of a well-intentioned but traditional sex therapist. Their recovery from shame, anxiety, and sexual aversion, and their acceptance of their non-erotic attachment, allowed each to pursue his or her own version of personal fulfillment. The couple regarded the treatment as a success.

COMMENTARY

There are no magic bullets for the cultural, political, psychological, social, or relational bases of sex problems. Adhering to a medical model that attempts to classify sexual problems as if they were in any way similar to medical disorders offers power to those who subscribe to prevailing cultural norms and disempowers those who see things differently. In the treatment of couples with sexual complaints, this can be harmful as well as unjust. Once ethical clinicians recognize that standards of sexual function and response change with the times, they then must avoid justifying standards and norms as if these represented clinical health rather than cultural power.

Arrangements about sexual frequency or passion are foremost matters of relational negotiation. The sex therapist as *therapist* unpacks motives and contributions of the past. Much about sex is reframed by the therapist as the patients are taught to challenge their assumptions along with those of the popular media (Tiefer, 2004). Most patients treated successfully gradually accept the perspective that beliefs and attitudes about sex are historical, negotiable, and flexible, and realize that such beliefs are asserted for rhetorical purposes rather than being statements of enduring fact. Without being didactic, the therapist illuminates the position that "being horny" is all about norms, in the same way as "dying for some chocolate" or "I have got to get some fresh air" are. These longings feel embodied and "purely" somatic and not at all cultural, but viewing them as having some noncultural source is not useful to therapy. The language of "sex drive" is avoided altogether. The sex therapist as *coach* facilitates sensual, recreational, emotional, and attitudinal learning and growth. The *ethical* therapist, mindful of misusing her authority, will not ally herself with cultural norms that insist sex is important to a successful relationship or with a mistaken medical model that links sexual conduct to mysterious but authoritarian notions of drive or libido. The desire to desire becomes one of many sociocultural topics under discussion as each case follows its unique trajectory.

REFERENCES

American Psychiatric Association. (1994). *Diagnostic and statistical manual of mental disorders* (4th ed.). Washington, DC: Author.

Brain, R. (1976). *Friends and lovers*. New York. Basic Books.

Chatterjee, C. (2001, September/October). Can men and women be friends? *Psychology Today, 34*, 61–67. Available at *www.psychologytoday.com/articles/pto-20010901-000031.html*.

Hall, M. (1998). *Lesbian love companion*. New York: HarperCollins.

Nye, R. A. (Ed.). (1999). *Sexuality*. New York: Oxford University Press.

Sexualityandu.ca. (2008). Life after puberty. Retrieved October 15, 2008, from *www.sexualityandu.ca/teens/life-5.aspx*.

Sprinkle, A. (1996). 101 uses for sex—or why sex is so important. *Women and Therapy, 19*(5–6). Excerpt on *www.anniesprinkle.org/html/writings/101_uses.html*.

Tiefer, L. (2004). *Sex is not a natural act and other essays*. Boulder, CO: Westview Press.

Tiefer, L. (2006). *The New View approach to men's sexual problems*. Retrieved October 15, 2008, from *www.medscape.com/viewprogram/5737_pnt*.

Working Group for a New View of Women's Sexual Problems. (2000). *A New View of women's sexual problems*. Retrieved October 15, 2008, from *www.newviewcampaign.org/manifesto.asp*.

Chapter 8

Complaints of Low Sexual Desire

How Therapeutic Assessment Guides Further Interventions

Rosemary Basson

In this chapter, Rosemary Basson highlights the many factors that contribute to sexual desire complaints in couples. Her case clearly illustrates the inherently relational aspects of sexual desire—the role of each partner in creating and maintaining sexual avoidance. Along with the developmental experiences and expectations of each partner that serve to subvert desire, one major precipitant, a husband's past extramarital affair and its discovery, seems to have set the stage for sexual avoidance by his wife. As Basson notes, this case illustrates the common observation that a woman's feelings for her partner most generally and especially at the time of sexual engagement, greatly influence sexual receptivity and interest.

Like many of the clinicians in this book, Basson emphasizes the necessity of treating both partners when there is a complaint of sexual dysfunction in either partner. One of the novel interventions in this case and in the one presented by her colleague, Lori A. Brotto in Chapter 9, is the inclusion of mindfulness training along with more traditional cognitive-behavioral and couple counseling interventions.

Finally, Basson emphasizes the current dilemma facing clinicians regarding androgen therapy. She clarifies the shortcomings of research studies that suggest that androgen deficiency underlies women's sexual desire/interest disorder and she proposes a more methodologically sound research approach.

Rosemary Basson, MD, is the Director of the Sexual Medicine Clinic at Vancouver General Hospital, as well as Clinical Professor in the Department of Psychiatry and the Department of Obstetrics and Gynecology at the University of British Columbia. Her reconceptualization of the sexual response cycle and her emphasis on the importance of arousal and motivation as critical components of sexual desire has had a major impact on the theory and treatment of women's sexual complaints.

The theoretical framework that guides my assessment and management of complaints of low sexual desire hinges on the concept that sexual motivation is larger than "desire" (as in drive or lust). The latter, often depicted as innate or even "spontaneous," normally lessens for women more so than it does for men as a relationship lengthens. The multitude of other reasons men and women engage in satisfying sex (Meston & Buss, 2007) motivates them to begin a sexual encounter even if desire is not the primary driving force on a particular occasion (and for some, women especially, on any recent occasion). There needs to be an expectation that desire will occur during the experience once pleasure and arousal are felt and the desire for more intense sexual sensation is triggered (see Figure 8.1). The expectation is that the desire so triggered will be enjoyable and appreciated by the partner.

Motivated, for example, by a need of emotional intimacy, appraisal of low-key sexual stimuli can lead to a degree of subjective arousal. If the required stimulation continues and the person attends to it, views it as both erotic and pleasurable, arousal intensifies, thereby triggering desire. This responsive desire invites stimuli that are considered by the person to be more intensely sexual: for instance, more purposeful genital stimulation. Arousal then becomes even more intense and a yearning for the physical as well as the emotional satisfaction of sex is now present. Orgasm(s) may or may not occur: for some people they are very important for their own satisfaction or for their partner's satisfaction. The subsequent well-being and emotional closeness that accompanies resolution of sexual sensations provides further motivation for future engagements. There is now qualitative research confirming the strong clinical impression that, for both men and women, arousal and desire are frequently not separable (Graham, Sanders & Milhausen, 2004; Janssen, McBride, Yarber, Hill, & Butler, 2008).

The sexual response cycle where a person starts from "neutral" is inherently vulnerable. Many psychological and some biological fac-

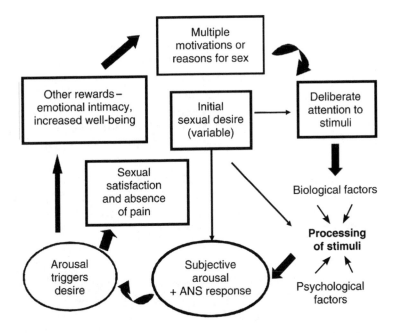

FIGURE 8.1. The sexual response cycle, a circular response cycle of overlapping phases: Desire may not be present initially but triggered during experience. The sexual and nonsexual outcome influences future sexual motivation. ANS, autonomic nervous system. Adapted from Basson (2001, Fig. 2). Copyright 2001 by the American College of Obstetricians and Gynecologists.

tors can limit the effectiveness of sexual stimuli. For women, their mood, their feelings for their partner generally and at the time of sexual interaction, and their ability to stay focused are major contributions to their experience of sexual desire and arousal. For men, these factors have received less research attention, although fear of performance failure or other negative outcomes appear to be common distractions (Bancroft & Janssen, 2000; Janssen et al., 2008).

Our clinic, the British Columbia Center for Sexual Medicine, located at Vancouver Hospital, British Columbia, Canada, receives relatively few referrals for hyperactive sexual desire other than in the context of neurological disease where "hypersexuality" must be distinguished from loss of inhibition. Other referrals are of men and women reporting excessive and often risky sexual activity as a means of coping with mood disturbance. Some ambivalence about giving up the "hunt" and the thrill of risk can hamper compliance with therapy.

Being a university-associated tertiary clinic, many of our referrals are for complicated erectile dysfunction, anejaculation, sexual pain, and sequelae of chronic neurological illness. Nevertheless, low desire is still the most prevalent concern in these and in our physically well patients. Usually the partner with low desire identifies as the patient but both partners are assessed and treated. When the "nonpatient" partner is reluctant or unwilling to attend sessions, the reason is usually a poor emotional relationship and the prognosis is also poor.

Challenges are many; frequently the issues are not strictly sexual despite the sexual symptoms, and in-depth psychotherapy is needed. For women, we now employ a small-group format for delivering therapy, which is a combination of cognitive-behavioral (CBT) interventions, sex therapy, sex education, and mindfulness techniques. Group treatment follows the initial assessment of the couple and has proven to be quite effective (Brotto, Basson, & Luria, 2008). To illustrate my approach to the treatment of low sexual desire, let me describe a recent case.

CASE EXAMPLE: TOM AND LUCY

Presenting Problem

Lucy and Tom are both 48 years old. Lucy presents saying "I just have no libido. If it was up to me it would be fine not ever to have sex again—I know this sounds terrible. It's not that I don't love Tom. I've never had much sexual drive but now it's zero." Tom adds, "You know, it isn't just Lucy. I think I am losing my desire too. We both feel that this is abnormal and both wish we were sexual more often."

The couple confirmed their marriage of 22 years was good and they were very fond of each other. They had many shared interests and there was no question of alcohol or substance abuse or any major current stresses at work or within the family. Their two sons were both doing well in college.

The couple explained that for Lucy's sake, they had saved intercourse for marriage, but nonpenetrative sex had been fine during their engagement of 3 years. Sex was described as rewarding, occurring perhaps weekly in the first number of years. They mentioned somewhat ruefully that they had never been a couple "who couldn't wait to rip each other's clothes off." Tom had always been the initiator but had frequently requested Lucy to do so. When seen privately in a subsequent session, Lucy recalled that she had initiated sex on one occasion but Tom was not interested. She found his refusal devastating and never tried initiating again.

Of note, until 5 years ago, Tom spent many weeks away from the home in his job as a mining engineer. When he was interviewed alone, it was clear that Tom did masturbate. In the past, he engaged in self-pleasuring some two to three times a week, more recently perhaps weekly.

He reported no concerns with his erection, ejaculation, or orgasm. He agreed his motivation to be sexual with Lucy was lessening and wondered if it was a reflection of her lessened interest and his needing it to be a mutually enjoyable experience; otherwise he saw no value in pursuing it.

In her individual interview, Lucy explained that she never had self-stimulated, being warned against it as a child. She had always felt awkward and shy about initiating sex. When sexual with Tom, Lucy was usually aroused and reported the experience to be pleasurable. Similarly, she was usually orgasmic with direct clitoral stimulation and reported no pain or discomfort with intercourse. She was puzzled as to why their sexual infrequency was so marked, given the frequently rewarding outcome. Often she asked herself, "Why don't we do this more often?"

The couple presented as affectionate and respectful. Lucy was particularly warm and outgoing, speaking very fondly of her partner, her family, and her work. Formerly a teacher in public schools, she now co-owns a private tutoring business. On each visit she arrived early and was perfectly dressed, manicured, and coiffed. Lucy agreed she liked to have herself and her life predictable and organized. Tom also came across as warm and generous, noncritical, supportive, and in no way blaming Lucy for their current predicament.

When seen separately, Tom admitted to an affair 10 years earlier. He said, "I'm not at all proud, I deeply regret it ever happening, I had just no idea it would ever be so devastating to Lucy." Lasting a few months, "it was pure sex." Tom had become enamored with a flirtatious mutual friend who apparently had very high sexual desire, and was very fond of initiating sex and very enthusiastic. Tom felt that his affair was still a relevant factor in their current sexual infrequency.

During Lucy's solo interview, she too mentioned the affair, describing how she became aware of the affair. She spoke of the severe shock it was to her. At the time she had been feeling very confident about herself. Her sons were then 8 and 10; she had more time for herself, had been working out, going to the gym, losing weight, and feeling attractive and confident. She felt she had just begun getting her life back, reentering the work force by forming a company with a friend for the private teaching of English as a second language. "Why did I not know it had been going on?"

Lucy's distress appeared to as be much about her inability to detect anything wrong or to be suspicious as about the affair/betrayal itself. Lucy explained that no particular counseling was given to the couple at the time. They briefly saw the local Roman Catholic priest, who said that these things happen rather commonly and that some good can come out of them. He even suggested that the marriage sometimes actually improves as a result. Lucy did not feel that the latter had happened. She explained how she had tried to make the very best of things and to be forgiving and as warm and affectionate as ever.

The couple have rarely addressed or spoken about the affair and its impact in any detail. Wanting to be more attractive to Tom, Lucy had very quickly found herself a plastic surgeon and received breast augmentation: she explained that the other woman had particularly large breasts whereas Lucy "was almost flat." Unfortunately, this led to loss of her former pleasurable nipple sexual sensitivity. Also Lucy was not pleased with the unnatural look and the excessive firmness. She has never sought revision but regrets her "foolish" decision to have the augmentation. Lucy spoke of her guilt that she must have been too preoccupied with the family or her new job, leading Tom to "stray."

Medical History

Tom was healthy and not taking any medications. Lucy's past medical history included having an imperforate hymen such that she presented with recurrent abdominal pain between the ages of 11 and 12 and had to be admitted to the hospital on an emergency basis for buildup of blood inside her uterus and pelvis. Additionally, as the result of a date rape at the age of 19, Lucy contracted genital herpes that was recurrent for a few years. The latter had not recurred during the pregnancies, to Lucy's huge relief. Each pregnancy had been marred by the fear herpes would harm their child. Lucy still saw herself as responsible for the date rape. At this time, however, Lucy was healthy with regular menses although she noted increasing mood lability and depressed thoughts premenstrually.

Developmental History: Lucy

Lucy reported that her childhood was chaotic. The family was Catholic; her father was an alcoholic and unfaithful to his wife. Lucy had little relationship with him. She did not fear him since he was not physically violent, even when drunk, but he was absent as a parent for her and her four siblings. The family moved many times and poverty was an ongoing problem. Her mother warned her repeatedly that sex would cause problems and definitely needed to be avoided until marriage. There were no positive messages about sex, either from her mother of from her Catholic school, where self-stimulation was described as sinful regardless of whether a person was single or married.

Developmental History: Tom

In describing his family history, Tom reported that his father was often away on business and Tom feared him when he was around as he had an unpredictable temper. His mother was described as aggressive and angry. At home, Tom stayed out of trouble by keeping a low profile, looking after his younger sisters, and being very responsible for them at a young age.

Tom says he never rebelled like other teen-agers: "that absolutely was not possible!" Puberty was normal and Tom reports only infrequent self-stimulation. He agrees that his sexuality has always been fairly low key. There were a couple of partners before Lucy and the sexual experiences were positive, but not particularly memorable or frequent.

Diagnoses

Tom was not diagnosed with any sexual disorder. Situational hypoactive sexual desire disorder (HSDD) was considered, but the only aspect of desire that was reduced was sex with Lucy: not only did self-stimulation continue, but sexual fantasies remained. His lessening frequency of self-stimulation was considered to be within normal limits for his age.

Lucy was diagnosed with DSM-IV HSDD. However, she could experience arousal and desire once sexually engaged. Therefore, she did not meet the diagnosis of sexual interest/desire disorder—a definition recommended by an international consensus committee in 2003 and endorsed by a larger international consensus committee representing major sexological and urological organizations in 2004 (Basson et al., 2004; Basson R., Brotto, L. A., Petkau, J., Labrie, F., in press).

Formulation

Part of Lucy's lack of sexual interest seemed related to the caution and negative messages she received about sex from her mother. Ironically, the warning that "sex will cause problems" was in some ways borne out: her sexual development as a teen was negative in a very dramatic way with the hematocolpos. In addition, the date rape followed a few years later, compounded by the distress of recurrent herpes. The lack of intensity in Tom's need to be sexual with her was another factor: although people can move on from the effects of negative themes about sex through childhood and adolescence, perhaps Tom's apparent lack of sexual intensity allowed Lucy to remain hesitant and never quite at peace with the idea of actually wanting sex.

Lucy's self-image was poor. She blamed herself for Tom's affair, for not being able to get over it, for her date rape, for potentially harming their babies should they have been affected by the herpes. As well, she claimed to have always been too thin and the breast augmentation had done little to improve her self-image. A major theme for Lucy was her need to be in control, which obviously served her well in getting through the chaos of her childhood, but it made the discovery of Tom's affair all the more devastating because she realized she was not in control of her life. Moreover, being in control is the antithesis of being sexual.

Precipitating factors for Lucy's lack of sexual desire included her reaction to Tom's affair. Although speaking initially of guilt, Lucy agreed that she had not dealt with her anger, feeling that anger was wrong. Suppressing her anger led to suppression of other emotions including sexual desire. Now, at midlife, hormonal changes might be implicated as well: midlife is associated with declining intracellular production of androgens. It is possible these changes were allowing the psychological issues to exert a greater impact.

In addition to the factors that may have precipitated the low sexual frequency between Tom and Lucy are the factors that maintained the status quo. These included Tom's rather low-key approach to sex, which is not uncommon in men from families in which self-assertion was not tolerated. Being assertive and being sexual are often linked: when one is suppressed, the other is often suppressed as well.

Tom agreed that he does not like to impose on others and not imposing sex on Lucy has been important for him. Sex during the affair was completely different. It was wonderful to be wanted sexually, but yet somewhat overwhelming. In retrospect Tom wonders if he would have eventually found it to be somewhat threatening. Being away from home so often because of his business may have contributed to Tom's reliance on self-stimulation. He acknowledged that masturbation is very different from partnered sex. The latter involved multiple reasons to go ahead or not and connected many emotions other than sexual ones, whereas, he added, "on my own it is very straightforward and easy and takes care of things."

Feedback to the Couple

The formulation was shared with the couple by explaining a model of the sexual response cycle. The composite cycle whereby there may or may not be desire initially in any one sexual experience, and arousal preceding and accompanying desire, was presented (see Figure 8.1). The various factors weakening Lucy's cycle were then identified.

1. Initiating /accepting invitations to sex. Lucy avoided initiating sex for reasons other than desire, such as to increase emotional closeness, due to her fear of rejection. At the beginning of their relationship, awkwardness, shyness, and even guilt about sex would also have precluded initiation. Mostly when Tom initiated Lucy accepted: the issue was that Tom did so infrequently.

2. The sexual context and stimuli were not always optimal. Late at night when sleep was needed was the usual timing.

3. There were many psychological factors that operated to decrease Lucy's arousal on those occasions when the sexual experience was unrewarding. Lucy's need to suppress her anger was one. It is very difficult to suppress just one emotion: all are likely to be suppressed, including sexual emotions. Low self-image was another, as was her discomfort with letting go of control.

4. Biological factors were not obvious. At age 48 Lucy may have up to 40% reduction of total testosterone production, but the relevance of this is quite unclear.

5. Although the outcome of being sexual together was frequently positive, it appeared not to motivate the couple to have a repeat experience. Lucy's fear of rejection and Tom's resentment that Lucy never

initiated prevailed. Also the times Lucy was not aroused left her with even less motivation to repeat the experience.

Treatment

Treatment involved a variety of interventions, including psychoeducation, CBT, sex therapy, and an introduction to mindfulness. Lucy declined a referral to a therapist in order to address her anger although she acknowledged that it was present.

Psychoeducation

The presentation and discussion of what was causing and maintaining their difficulty was itself therapeutic. Both partners expressed relief at having some understanding of why each was sexually hesitant. They especially appreciated learning how each partner enabled the other to stay the same.

Cognitive-Behavioral Therapy

Having briefly discussed the various reasons men and women have sex, the couple filled out forms checking reasons they might or might not initiate or agree to sex. Lucy found this difficult because, as she said, "I never initiate," but she was able to see the value in identifying some of the items that hold her back from making a sexual overture to Tom. She was encouraged to make thought records of some of these misgivings and discovered many of them were overstated if not catastrophic. More balanced evidence-based thoughts were encouraged.

Tom realized that in addition to holding back because he resented Lucy's failure to initiate sex, he needed to see Lucy's enjoyment and sexual excitement. Without Lucy's excitement his own arousal required total absorption in his own sexual fantasies. Were he to do this when making love to Lucy he felt that he would be unfaithful all over again. He was encouraged to consider whether he truly believed his fantasizing was equivalent to being unfaithful.

Behavioral interventions included making several practical changes, such as the use of low lighting so that Tom could see Lucy during sex, as well as beginning sexual engagements earlier in the day so as to avoid the battle between fatigue and arousal.

Small-Group Therapy for Lucy

In addition to the interventions described, Lucy attended four 2-hour small-group sessions held 2 weeks apart and led by two therapists. Sexual response cycles were discussed, clarifying that most women in long-term relationships have sex for reasons other than desire, at least at the outset. Also emphasized was the importance of context—interpersonal and environmental, as well as cultural contexts, were also outlined. That women frequently have difficulty staying focused and being present in the moment was acknowledged and led directly into discussion of the technique of mindfulness. In their sessions the group discussed and practiced cultivating a state of "relaxed wakefulness" whereby the goal is to remain in the moment and ultimately to observe distracting thoughts but not follow them. Daily practice of mindfulness was encouraged.

The cognitive work included identifying inaccurate and catastrophic thoughts about sexuality, attractiveness, and worthiness. Thought records were described and encouraged. Lucy and the other women completed assignments between the sessions that involved both the cognitive work and the mindfulness practice. Further assignments involved encouraging communication and listening skills.

Therapy for Tom

Tom said he had been intrigued by the possible connection between his coping skills in childhood and his low-key sexuality as an adult. He was interested in becoming more assertive in appropriate circumstances outside of the bedroom. It was suggested that being flexible might be more helpful than always being nonassertive.

After Lucy completed the four group therapy sessions, the couple was seen again and a modified sensate focus program over 3 weeks was outlined. Lucy was encouraged to continue the mindfulness practice; the similarities between the two therapies were obvious.

Outcome

When Tom and Lucy were seen 3 months later, each described more rewarding sexual encounters. Lucy was still hesitant about initiating sex with Tom. Their sexual frequency had increased somewhat. Though she was far less distressed about her situation, Lucy still mourned her absent libido. Again the idea of brief psychotherapy to address her anger was raised, and this time Lucy accepted.

Seen again 2 months later, Lucy spoke of the relief of finally losing "her burden." She felt free to be herself and was no longer checking or censoring herself. She had decided to risk initiating sex and allow her feelings to be apparent should Tom decline. So far Tom had shown no intention of refusing her invitations!

THE ROLE OF DECLINING ANDROGEN PRODUCTION

For men, if serum testosterone levels drop sufficiently low, desire decreases, sexual fantasies cease, and self-stimulation becomes infrequent or stops altogether. As serum testosterone levels reduce and the man attempts sexual activity, there is delay in ejaculation, minimal ejaculate, and non-intense orgasm. Nocturnal erections stop as well. Sexually stimulated erections may still occur if there are adequate visual stimuli.

For women, there is no correlation sexual testosterone levels, however measured, and sexual function. Two major confounds have hampered conclusions regarding women's sexual function and the role of androgens. First, until recently, serum assays have been extremely unreliable and insensitive because of the low level of testosterone found in women. Now, at least in research settings, mass spectrometry is available and accurate. Perhaps most important, the percentage of testosterone produced but never entering the circulation to be measured is high in women although very low in men. At least 50% of younger women's testosterone is derived from precursor hormones, namely, dehydroepiandrosterone (DHEA), DHEA sulfate, androstenedione from the adrenal glands, and DHEA and androstenedione from the ovaries. Androgen metabolites—most notably androsterone glucuronide (ADTG)—reflect the total androgen production (Labrie et al., 2006). Our clinic is collaborating with Professor Fernand Labrie in Quebec, who has developed the assays for the metabolite measurement: we have not identified any correlation between androgen metabolites and women's sexual function (Basson et al., in press).

Although surgical menopause has been cited as an example of androgen deficiency, the prevalence of subsequent loss of sexual desire and arousal is unknown. Cross-sectional studies of women with surgical menopause report more distress over low desire and low satisfaction than do naturally postmenopausal women. However, prospective studies of sexual outcome after elective bilateral oophorectomy along with required simple hysterectomy fail to show subsequent sexual dysfunction (Aziz, Brannstrom, Bergquist, & Silfverstolper, 2005; Farquar, Harvey, Yu, Sadler, & Stewart, 2006; Teplin et al., 2007). Aside from any loss of ovarian production of testosterone or its precursor hormones, adrenal production of precursors is thought to decrease by some 70% between the mid-30s and the late 60s. However the amount of variation among individual women is unknown; decreased production in some women may still be sufficient if the necessary enzymes in the cells that convert the precursors to testosterone and estrogen remain sufficiently active. Measurement of androgen metabolites reflects not only the level of substrate, that is, the precursor hormones, but the ability of the enzymes to convert them. However, there is still a large caveat to this: this measure of androgen metabolites will still not account for any variation in sensitivity of the androgen receptor and the availability of co-factors. Moreover there may be an even more important confound, namely the fact that the brain can synthesize sex hormones from the basic building block of cholesterol (King, 2008). Additionally, there is some evidence that after menopause this intracerebral production of neurosteroids increases (Ishunina & Swaab, 2007).

Despite these difficulties in correlating women's sexual function with androgen activity, in some countries outside North America transdermal testosterone has been approved for women with a DMS-IV diagnosis of HSDD subsequent to surgical menopause. There is major concern about the lack of long-term safety studies. Somewhat ironically, women are often denied estrogen therapy postmenopause on the basis of the Women's Health Initiative study, which showed increased harm when estrogen is begun 10 or so years after menopause. This decision to avoid estrogen therapy continues despite the fact that the younger women closer to menopause showed benefit rather than harm (Hodis & Mack, 2008). Women and their clinicians are understandably very confused that with very limited data systemic testosterone has been approved elsewhere and is given off label in North America, while simultaneously estrogen is denied to women whose histories suggest that they are in the subgroup of women who would benefit. The transdermal testosterone approval has been for estrogenized women only. A recent study showed benefit to estrogen-deficient women with HSDD who are naturally menopausal; those who were surgically menopausal did not benefit. Another recent study showed minimal benefit from transdermal testosterone when given to premenopausal women with HSDD.

Of major importance is the omission from all of these trials of women with sexual interest/desire disorder (Basson, 2008). All recruited women were reporting two to three satisfying sexual engagements per month at baseline. Women with sexual interest/desire disorder report no satisfying events, as desire and arousal cannot be triggered during the experience.

CASE EXAMPLE, CONTINUED: LUCY'S ANDROGEN METABOLITES

As part of our ongoing study of androgen metabolites and women's sexual function, Lucy agreed to complete questionnaires on her own sexual function and have a blood sample taken for androgen metabolites. The results showed values at the high end of the normal range for the women of her age.

COMMENTARY

Lucy and Tom's story reflects some of the common themes present when one or both partners complain of low desire. First, sexual function and dysfunction are inherently relational. Tom's relative sexual passivity enabled Lucy's misgivings about sex to continue. Lucy never felt that Tom was passionate about her. His affair further undermined her low sexual self-image. Lucy's preference for sex in the dark at bedtime enabled Tom's style of "sex alone" to continue. Without seeing his partner, Tom resorted to his own sexual fantasies but then felt he was again being unfaithful. Thus, he avoided sex with Lucy even more.

This case also illustrates the common finding that women's feelings for the partner generally and at the time of sexual engagement correlate highly with their desire. For Lucy her feelings for Tom were still marred by the nonresolution of her feelings surrounding his affair.

When we consider which women complain about their low desire, we are reminded that even when a diagnosis of clinical depression is excluded, women who report low desire have been shown to have more anxious and depressed thoughts, more mood lability, and lower self-esteem than control women (Hartmann, Philippsohn, Heiser, & Ruffer-Hesse, 2004). Lucy's self-image improved somewhat from the CBT approach in the group therapy but more so from the brief psychotherapy where she allowed herself to feel and express her anger about Tom's affair and receive support for having those feelings rather than continuing with her self-condemnation.

The major helpful intervention in this case was explaining the logic of the woman's situation to Lucy and Tom (Basson, 2008). Learning that they were reacting "normally" given their childhood experiences, their past sexual history, and the current context rather than being "broken" sexually was immensely therapeutic. Women, especially, feel more competent sexually once they are reassured that they are not sexually deficient. The CBT aspect of the group session helped Lucy to identify negative and catastrophic thoughts and to change them. Finally, the introduction of mindfulness practice allowed Lucy to realize that the times she was not aroused were times when she was not mentally present. Only with continued mindfulness practice will distractions be less damaging, but the recognition that the constant chatter in her mind precluded arousal and pleasure was comforting. This case also illustrates the power of unresolved anger and the need to address it.

REFERENCES

Aziz, A., Brannstrom, M., Bergquist, C., & Silfverstolper, G. (2005). Perimenopausal androgen decline after oophorectomy does not influence sexuality or psychological well-being. *Fertility and Sterility, 83,* 1021–1028.

Bancroft, J., & Janssen, E. (2000). The dual control model of male sexual response: A theoretical approach to centrally mediated erectile dysfunction. *Neuroscience and Biobehavioral Reviews, 24,* 571–579.

Basson, R. (2001). Female sexual response: The role of drugs in the management of sexual dysfunction. *Obstetrics and Gynecology, 98*(2), 350–352.

Basson, R. (2008). Women's sexual desire and arousal disorders. *Primary Psychiatry, 15,* 72–81.

Basson, R., Brotto, L. A., Petkau, J., Labrie, F. (in press). Role of androgens in women's sexual dysfunction. *Menopause.*

Basson, R., Leiblum, S., Brotto, L., Derogatis, L., Fourcroy, J., & Fugl-Meyer, K. (2004). Revised definitions of women's sexual dysfunction. *Journal of Sexual Medicine, 1,* 40–48.

Brotto, L. A., Basson, R., & Luria, M. (2008). A mindfulness-based group psychoeducational intervention targeting sexual arousal disorder in women. *Journal of Sexual Medicine, 1,* 40–48.

Brotto, L. A., Bitzer, J., Laan, E., Leiblum, S., Luria, M. (in press). Women's sexual desire and arousal disorders. *Journal of Sexual Medicine.*

Farquhar, C. M., Harvey, S. A., Yu, Y., Sadler, L., & Stewart, A. W. (2006). A prospective study of 3 years of outcomes after hysterectomy with and without oophorectomy. *American Journal of Obstetrics and Gynecology, 194,* 711–717.

Graham, C. A., Sanders, S. A., Milhausen, R. R., & McBride, K. R. (2004). Turning on and turning off: A focus group study of the factors that affect women's sexual arousal. *Archives of Sexual Behavior, 33,* 527–538.

Hartmann, U., Philippsohn, S., Heiser, K., & Ruffer-Hesse, C. (2004). Low sexual desire in midlife and older women: Personality factors, psychosocial development, present sexuality. *Menopause, 11,* 726–740.

Hodis, H. N., & Mack, W. J. (2008). Postmenopausal hormone therapy and cardiovascular disease in perspective. *Clinical Obstetrics and Gynecology, 51,* 564–580.

Ishunina, T. A., & Swaab, D. F. (2007). Alterations in the human brain in menopause. *Maturitas, 57,* 20–22.

Janssen, E., McBride, K. R., Yarber, W., Hill, B. J., & Butler, S. M. (2008). Factors that influence sexual arousal in men: A focus group study. *Archives of Sexual Behavior, 37,* 252–265.

King, S. R. (2008). Emerging roles for neurosteroids in sexual behavior and function. *Journal of Andrology, 29,* 524–533.

Labrie, F., Belanger, A., Belanger, P., Berube, R., Martel, C., & Cusan, L. (2006). Androgen glucuronides, instead of testosterone, as the new markers of androgenic activity in women. *Journal of Steroid Biochemistry and Molecular Biology, 99,* 182–188.

Meston, C. M., & Buss, D. M. (2007). Why humans have sex. *Archives of Sexual Behavior, 36,* 477–507.

Teplin, V., Vittinghoff, E., Lin, F., Learman, L. A., Richter, H. E., & Kuppermann, M. (2007). Oophorectomy in premenopausal women: Health-related quality of life and sexual functioning. *Obstetrics and Gynecology, 109,* 347–354.

Chapter 9

Cognitive-Behavioral and Mindfulness-Based Therapy for Low Sexual Desire

Lori A. Brotto
Jane S. T. Woo

In this chapter, Lori A. Brotto and Jane S. T. Woo illustrate the additional benefits of adding a mindfulness component to more traditional cognitive-behavioral treatment of low desire. The authors suggest that mindfulness is particularly helpful for those women and men who are given to distraction and/or distressing negative automatic thoughts during sexual activity. By learning to be aware of their thoughts in a nonjudgmental way, such patients can not only learn to be fully present and alert to their sexual arousal, but also to understand that thoughts are just thoughts and are not necessarily accurate representations of reality.

In the case presented, treatment interventions are focused on the "identified" patient, the woman who feels guilty and deficient about her lack of desire and who tends to be self-critical and easily distracted from her own sensual experience. The additional component of a four-session short-term small-group intervention along with mindfulness training appears to be quite helpful in reinforcing the learning that occurs during therapy.

Lori A. Brotto, PhD, is Assistant Professor in the Department of Obstetrics and Gynaecology at the University of British Columbia. Her research focuses largely on testing psychoeducational interventions for women with various forms of sexual dysfunction (e.g., low desire, arousal, vestibulodynia). Dr. Brotto is on the Sexual Dysfunctions subworkgroup for DSM-V.

Jane S. T. Woo, MA, is a doctoral candidate in Clinical Psychology at the University of British Columbia. Her research is focused on Asian women's sexuality and barriers to reproductive health testing.

Problems in sexual desire are the most frequent complaint in every population-based and clinical study conducted on women. The prevalence of low desire with distress ranges anywhere from 8 to 26%, depending on the study, the country, and the methodology. In the clinical practice setting in which we work—a tertiary care hospital-based sexual medicine clinic—low sexual desire in women is the most frequent presenting complaint. The challenge in treating desire cases—whether the identified patient is male or female—is the comorbidity of low desire with other issues such as mood disorders, anxiety, fatigue, acute and/or chronic health problems, medications, inadequate nutrition, demands of parenting, work-associated stress, financial issues, poor body image, insufficient or inaccurate knowledge about genital anatomy and physiology, and poor dyadic communication. Other challenges include the level of insight and motivation of the woman and her partner. It is not uncommon for patients to present with the expectation that problems can be identified and resolved in a few short sessions. Misconceptions about treatment are common, and patients may be disappointed to learn that there will be no "quick fix" for restoring their sexual motivation.

The challenge of untangling the many issues associated with desire cases is further complicated when problems have been present for many years, with the resulting layers of resentment, guilt, frustration, and anxiety. In our clinic, women often describe their loss of or absent desire in any number of ways including: "I don't care about sex," "I only have sex to please my partner," "I'd rather do laundry then have sex," and so on.

HOW TO DEFINE DESIRE

There are varying definitions of sexual desire disorder in the clinical research literature. In the current edition of the *Diagnostic and Statistical Manual of Mental Disorders* (DSM-IV-TR), hypoactive sexual desire disorder (HSDD) is defined as "persistently or recurrently deficient (or absent) sexual fantasies and desire for sexual activity." It is interesting to note that women rarely (if ever) present with the complaint of lack of sexual fantasies. In the definition proposed by an international consensus committee in 2003, women's sexual desire /interest disorder is defined as "absent or diminished feelings of sexual interest or desire, absent sexual thoughts or fantasies and a lack of responsive desire." This definition suggests that it is the lack of "responsive desire," or desire to continue the sexual encounter once some excitement is reached, that is a better indicator of a desire problem.

Validated questionnaires also define sexual desire in slightly different ways. For example, in the Sexual Interest and Desire Inventory, sexual desire is captured by a number of different items, including receptivity to and initiation of sexual activity, wanting sexual activity, thinking about sex, and responsive sexual desire. In the Sexual Desire Inventory, sexual desire is conceptualized with a focus on the cognitive domain and is defined as "interest in sexual activity. It [desire] is primarily a cognitive variable, which can be measured through the amount and strength of thought directed toward approaching or being responsive to sexual stimuli."

It is evident from these examples that sexual desire may be conceptualized and operationalized quite differently. When women themselves are asked how they define desire, their definitions are even more varied, with some expressing confusion about what desire is or conflation between the terms desire and arousal. Desire may be viewed as a cognitive experience (e.g., thoughts or fantasies; motivations), an emotional entity (e.g., feelings of sexual interest, wanting sexual activity), or a behavioral event (e.g., receptivity to or initiation of sexual activity), with the different questionnaires and definitions emphasizing the cognitive, emotional, and behavioral elements to varying degrees. To illustrate how these three dimensions may manifest themselves, consider the example of a woman who reports avoiding going to bed at the same time as her partner (i.e., behavior) given her belief that he will request sexual activity (i.e., cognition) resulting in her feeling frustrated that she is "not in the mood" and resentful that he has the energy to devote to sex whereas she feels utterly exhausted (i.e., emotions). (See Figure 9.1.) Thus, this conceptualization lends itself well to cognitive-behavioral treatment interventions.

What Is Cognitive-Behavioral Therapy?

Cognitive-behavioral therapy (CBT) is a form of psychotherapy that emphasizes the interconnections among cognitions, emotions, and behaviors. The CBT model suggests that changing any one of these three components leads to changes in the others. Treatment for emotional difficulties targets cognitions and behaviors as a pathway to moderate emotions. CBT emerged from the synthesis of the radical behaviorism of the 1950s with cognitive therapy and was heavily influenced by the work of Beck (1993) and Ellis (1962), who regarded irrational thoughts and faulty cognitive processing as the source of emotional distress.

CBT has been applied to the treatment of numerous mental disorders including mood disorders, anxiety disorders, schizophrenia, eating disorders, and personality disorders, and has received consistent empirical support for its efficacy. In the domain of female sexual disorders, CBT has been shown to be efficacious for orgasmic disorder, vaginismus, and some types of dyspareunia.

To date, only two studies have explored the efficacy of CBT in the treatment of low sexual desire. In an uncontrolled study, McCabe (2001) examined the utility of CBT in treating men and women with various sexual dysfunctions. The 10-session treatment program consisted of exercises designed to improve communication between partners, enhance sexual skills, decrease sexual and performance anxiety, and alter cognitions and behaviors that interfered with these domains. Of the 43 women who complained of lack of sexual interest and who completed the treatment program, 33% reported that treatment was helpful. Trudel and colleagues (2001) randomly assigned 74 couples in which the female partner had low sexual desire to either a CBT treatment group or a 3-month waitlist group. Following treatment (12 weekly group couple therapy sessions plus homework), CBT was helpful for 74% of women, and 64% of the women maintained their gains after 1 year.

What follows is a case example illustrating the use of CBT with a middle-aged couple.

CASE EXAMPLE: MONA AND HARRY

Presenting Complaint

Mona, 49, and Harry, 56, who have been married for 20 years, presented for treatment with the primary complaint of infrequent sexual intercourse. Mona is a premenopausal woman who owns her own fashion design company and Harry is a manager of a busy factory. They have one 10-year old son. They described once-monthly sexual activity, occurring late at night. Typically, Harry would ask Mona if they could have sex and she would reluctantly agree. They described minimal to no foreplay, consisting of a few minutes of kissing followed immediately by sexual intercourse.

During sexual activity, Mona said that her mind was focused on wondering when sex would be over. She reported thinking about work or the many items on her to-do list. She described herself as a multitasker in the rest of her life as well, during which she found it difficult to stay focused on one task at a time. She also feared their son would hear her and as a result requested that Harry keep his sounds of pleasure to a minimum. She reported having desire "out of the blue" approximately once a month during ovulation, but she did not seek out Harry during these times nor did she ever masturbate. Mona reported only a minimal genital arousal response during sex, and denied ever having an orgasm in her life. However, intercourse was not painful. She indicated that she has never really craved sexual activity, but that her current absence of any desire has been especially pronounced for at least 10 years, since the birth of their son and the death of her father at about the same time.

Prior to seeking treatment, Mona and Harry had tried a few different sexual positions (at Harry's suggestion) in hopes of creating more pleasure. They had also tried a course of AndroGel (50 mg), which she applied to her abdomen four hours before sexual activity, prescribed by Mona's family physician. Neither of these interventions was helpful. Their current request for treatment was prompted by Harry's increasing frustration at their infrequent sexual activity, which was creating tension in their relationship. Whereas their communication, in general, was very good, the topic of sexuality made Mona anxious and she retreated to her office when Harry wanted to discuss sex.

Assessment

During her individual interview, Mona described a dislike of sexual activity and embarrassment about sexual topics. She avoided clitoral touch and did not allow Harry to touch her genitals. Mona had had a few boyfriends prior to Harry, but he was her first sexual partner. Within 6 months of meeting they began to have sexual intercourse. For Mona this was accompanied by significant guilt—she believed that she should remain a virgin until marriage. To this day, she reported still carrying guilt whenever she was sexual. Religious reasons also prevented her from ever trying to masturbate, stemming from her belief that masturbation is a sin. Mona did have nocturnal orgasms though she kept this information private.

In terms of psychiatric status, Mona had experienced one major depressive episode following the death of her father 10 years ago. It coincided with a bout of postpartum depressive symptoms. Presently, her mood was good though she was prone to anxiety and occasional panic attacks. She described having a hard time relaxing, which was difficult for Harry, who enjoys spending time away from work watching movies or taking naps. She denied any history of childhood or adult sexual abuse.

During his individual interview, Harry stated that he feared his sexual desire was abnormally high as he desired sex every day. Prior to meeting Mona, he had had 15 different sexual partners. He desperately wanted to please Mona but she was highly resistant to his efforts. Harry reported being firmly committed to Mona and although he was tempted to have an extramarital affair, he would not. He thought that Mona's low desire was attributable to her strong Christian faith, which precluded premarital intercourse. He also worried about Mona's distractibility—he could sense that her mind was elsewhere when they made love. He described this experience as feeling like he was having sex with a robot.

Mona's health was excellent. She exercised regularly and did not smoke or consume alcohol. She was not using any medications, although she did suffer from migraine headaches (once a month) for which she used Tylenol 3 with adequate effectiveness. She had no history of endocrine problems and her surgical history included appendectomy and tonsillectomy at the ages of 17 and 19, respectively.

Following their conjoint and then individual interviews, Mona took part in an investigational hormone assessment as part of a larger research trial. This involved assaying a small sample of her serum for testosterone metabolites and precursors (e.g., dehydroepiandrosterone and dihydrotestosterone), as well as mass spectrometry analyses of free testosterone and estradiol. The results of her androgen metabolites and precursors, estradiol, and testosterone were all in the normal range for women in their 40s and 50s.

Formulation

Mona did not have sexual thoughts, fantasies, or desire for sexual activity. She did not want sexual stimulation to continue when actively engaging in sex even when her body started to show signs of physical arousal. Thus, she met criteria for both the DSM-IV definition of HSDD and for sexual desire/interest disorder, as defined by the International Consensus Committee, focusing on lack of responsive desire. On the basis of her medical history, her premenopausal status, and the results from her androgen metabolites, it is unlikely that there was a significant medical and/or hormonal component to Mona's reduced sexual desire.

Mona had several problematic automatic thoughts. Among them was the belief that her son might hear them having sex, masturbation was wrong, and it was inappropriate for Harry to touch her genitals. Mona had sex solely out of a sense of obligation, she resented being asked for sex by Harry, and she experienced guilt for not making it enjoyable for Harry. Her behaviors included avoidance of talking about her low desire, deliberately going to bed after Harry, and thinking about other obligations on her to-do list during sex. Each of these cognitions, emotions, and behaviors led to a cascade of other thoughts, feelings, and behaviors; thus, a tightly woven vicious circle was spun around Mona's sexual activity and low desire.

A CBT approach seemed indicated for Mona in light of her core beliefs, which resulted in her emotional and behavioral difficulties. Such a treatment would focus on identifying, challenging, and replacing her automatic thoughts related to sex. It was helpful for Mona to complete a thought–feeling–behavior form (Figure 9.1) to see the range of her automatic thoughts and how they gave rise to a host of negative emotions and problematic behaviors. She was given instruction to use a blank CBT diagram and to fill in her thoughts, feelings, and behaviors during a recent negative sexual interaction with her partner. However, given Mona's significant distractibility, multitasking, and anxiety proneness, a mindfulness-based cognitive-behavioral intervention seemed important to add.

WHAT IS MINDFULNESS?

Mindfulness is the practice of intentionally being fully aware of one's thoughts, emotions, and physical sensations in a nonjudgmental way. Although mindfulness is rooted in Eastern spiritual practices, it is rapidly being embraced in Western approaches to both physical and mental health care. Mindfulness-based treatments have been found to have therapeutic benefits in disorders ranging from pain to depres-

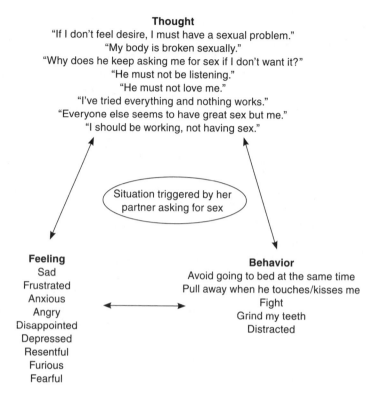

FIGURE 9.1. Thought–feeling–behavior form.

sion, anxiety disorders, eating disorders, substance abuse, and borderline personality disorder.

Mindfulness has been referred to as the third wave in the evolution of behavior-based therapies, with the first phase (behavior therapy) characterized by an exclusive focus on correcting problematic behaviors and the second (CBT) defined by the inclusion of irrational thoughts and faulty cognitive processing as additional treatment targets. Mindfulness complements CBT by providing additional tools with which to understand the phenomenological experience of their thoughts and feelings. By teaching patients to be aware of their thoughts in a nonjudgmental way, for instance, the experience of mindfulness leads patients to understand that thoughts are just thoughts and are not necessarily accurate representations of reality.

MINDFULNESS-BASED TREATMENTS AND SEXUALITY

The literature testing mindfulness for sexual problems is limited to two studies from our group as well as one qualitative study in nondistressed couples. Among the latter, a mindfulness-based intervention significantly enhanced relationship satisfaction and reduced distress (Carson, Carson, Gil, & Baucom, 2004). In a study of women who were treated for cervical or endometrial cancer, a brief individual psychoeducational intervention (PED) with mindfulness as one of its core components led to significantly improved sexual desire, arousal, orgasm, and satisfaction (Brotto et al., 2008). Importantly, sexuality-related distress and depressive symptoms also decreased. Qualitative analyses of women's experience during the PED revealed that the mindfulness component was seen as most helpful because it helped women become aware of residual genital arousal that they believed had been lost by virtue of their prior surgery. Attending to these sensations further enhanced their subjective excitement.

Following the positive findings of the PED group in the first study, we studied a population of women with sexual arousal and desire complaints unrelated to cancer. The general interventions remained the same, although the PED was administered in a group format. The results revealed an increase in self-reported sexual desire and a decrease in sexuality-related distress. In particular, those women with a history of sexual assault and who were therefore prone to distraction during sexual activity responded especially positively (Brotto, Basson, & Luria, 2008).

CASE EXAMPLE, CONTINUED

Treatment

Following the initial two assessment sessions, Mona took part in four 90-minute group sessions, which combined elements of education, cognitive and behavioral skills, and mindfulness practice. Education focused on a discussion of the definition of sexual desire and arousal, provided her with available epidemiological data on the prevalence of sexual difficulties, and discussed aspects of female genital anatomy and physiology. The latter was particularly helpful for Mona, who had never "explored" her own genitals and was unaware of the rich vasculature of the clitoris and vestibular bulbs.

The CBT elements of treatment involved a detailed discussion and illustration of the cognitive-behavioral model, using an example from Mona's own experience to illustrate the vicious cycle of thoughts, feelings, and behaviors (see Figure 9.1). Mona took home and completed thought records to track the frequency and intensity of her irrational beliefs and to form new balanced thoughts to replace them (see Figures 9.2 and 9.3). She benefitted from hearing other women normalize aspects of their own sexual experience, and after four sessions, Mona was able to allow Harry to touch her without the previous experience of anxiety and belief that this was wrong. She also began to identify and challenge her own avoidance behavior as she now realized the role of avoidance in perpetuating her anxiety and low desire.

The mindfulness exercises were varied and extensive and involved in-session practice as well as daily practice between ses-

---

A thought record can be an effective way of identifying negative thoughts, understanding their link with particularly strong emotions, and challenging and replacing them with more balanced (or rational) thoughts. When you have a strong emotion (e.g., anger, sadness, resentment, guilt, frustration), this can be a clue that there are automatic (and negative) thoughts present. For this exercise, we would like you to practice tracking your automatic thoughts for 1 week. When you have a strong emotion, document the emotion and how intense it is on a scale of 0–10 in column 1. Note the day and time and the situation that triggered it in column 2. Then, try to identify in column 3 what are the automatic thoughts underlying or associated with that emotion. In column 4 write how strongly (from 1 to 10) you believed that thought. Columns 5 and 6 are where you collect the evidence for and against the particular thoughts listed in column 3.

Some questions to ask yourself to help find evidence against your automatic thought are:

- "Have I had any experiences that would suggest this thought is not true all the time?"
- "If my best friend or someone I loved had this thought, what would I tell them?"
- "When I am not feeling this way, would I think about this type of situation differently?"
- "When I have felt this way in the past, what did I do or think about to make myself feel better?"
- "Are there any small things that contradict my thoughts that I might be discounting as not important?"
- "Am I jumping to conclusions with my automatic thoughts?"
- "Am I blaming myself for something over which I do not have complete control?"

If your exercise in collecting the evidence does not support your automatic thought, then in column 7 write an alternative or balanced view of the situation that is consistent with the evidence. Then, in column 8, rate your belief in the balanced thought, any change in your mood, and the outcome.

FIGURE 9.2. Thought record instructions.

Emotion How did you feel? (0–10)	Situation Who? What? Where? When?	Automatic thought(s) What exactly were your thoughts?	Strength of thought How strongly do you believe this thought (0–10)?	Evidence supporting the automatic thought	Evidence not supporting the automatic thought	Alternative or balanced thoughts	Outcome How much do you believe the balanced thoughts (0–10)? How do you now feel (0–10)? What can you do?
Angry (3) Anxious (7) Resentful (5)	Husband came up behind me while I was on the computer and placed his hand on my back.	"He must not love me if he keeps asking for sex."	(9)	He touched my back—an intimate part.	Touching my back is not the same as asking for sex. He shows me he loves me. He tells me he loves me. I've never told him not to touch my back. I'm tired and thinking emotionally.	Touching my back is a sign of affection, not necessarily a request for sex. My husband does love me.	Balanced thought: 10 Old thought: 2

FIGURE 9.3. A thought record in response to one specific negative thought evoked when anticipating sexual activity.

159

sions. Mona first took part in a nonsexual exercise in session that involved exploring, sensing, and tasting a raisin in great detail. She was given the instruction to "take in" this raisin—to drink it with her eyes and to bring her mind back to the present should she be distracted, and to resist judging herself should her mind wander. In doing this nonsexual exercise, Mona realized just how distractible she was. However, she also learned that she could guide her attention into the present moment if she chose to do so. This was very rewarding for Mona to realize given her prior belief that her brain was "wired" only to multitask. She then practiced a 30-minute body scan four times per week, which involved mindfully noticing the different parts of her body and breathing diaphragmatically into those parts. With practice she became more aware of what triggers led to distraction.

Mona next began to practice mindfulness exercises involving her own body. She was asked to take a bath or shower and mindfully be aware of her skin as she dried—not spending time on the negative judgments that would inevitably come up. Mona learned to remain focused in the present and to squelch such judgments. She practiced a mindfulness exercise while visually exploring her own genitals with the aid of a diagram and handheld mirror, and secondly with the use of her own fingers. She found these exercises difficult as she strongly associated genital touch with guilt. However, she was able to redirect her mind into the present and enjoyed learning about her genitals, which ultimately resulted in reduced anxiety with genital touch.

We then practiced a mindfulness exercise in which she first attempted to adopt a positive sexual self-schema (e.g., she read a paragraph indicating to her that she enjoyed her own sexuality, and she was feminine and sensual). With this cognitive schema in mind, Mona practiced the body scan exercise. Although she did not believe the schema stating that she enjoyed her sexuality, she could adopt it temporarily during these practice sessions. Another component of the mindfulness exercises involved encouraging Mona to utilize fantasy, erotica, and/or vibrators as a means of boosting sexual arousal. This was a challenging exercise for Mona given her resistance to these tools and view of them as being inappropriate. However, we conceptualized them as sexual aids to be used in a very specific way. After experiencing some arousal after a few minutes of either imagining a fantasy about herself and Harry, watching some "female-friendly" erotica, or using a personal massager on her genitals, Mona was to then discontinue this and immediately do a body scan for 15 minutes. The rationale was given that by first exciting her mind (through fantasy) or body (through erotica or vibrator), this would increase the chances that her mind and body could remain in sync through mindfulness.

Therapy Outcome

The combination of mindfulness and CBT was ideally suited for Mona. CBT allowed her to identify, challenge, and replace many of the automatic (and irrational) thoughts she had about sexuality. It also allowed her to understand the role that avoidance behavior played in maintaining her resentment of Harry and in perpetuating her low desire. The detailed thought records completed by Mona (Figure 9.3) allowed her to see the delicate interactions between her thoughts, feelings, and behaviors so that she could predict ahead of time how having a particular thought might lead her to feel bad or avoid interactions with Harry. They also encouraged her to adopt new, balanced thoughts to replace irrational beliefs.

Mindfulness directly targeted her distractibility and judgmental tendencies. Mona believed at the outset that her mind was naturally wired to be in many different places at one time. She never challenged this during any activity, for she perceived it as beneficial to "accomplish" many things at the same time. However, this meant that during sexual activity she was focused on other, nonsexual events that were more pressing. Mona accepted the rationale of mindfulness in session. The fact that mindfulness has been found to result in structural and functional changes in the brain provided for Mona the necessary evidence to immerse herself completely in the exercises. By beginning our practice in nonsexual situations, Mona was able to hone her practice and start to enjoy the experience of being in the moment throughout various activities in her day. Mona found that practicing mindful exercises with her own body was more challenging (as most women do), given that an array of body-specific negative judgments were triggered. She realized that she was a highly judgmental person—of herself and of Harry—and began to wonder how much her judgmental style led her to be naturally resentful of Harry. When the mindfulness exercises were eventually paired with some sexually arousing activities (e.g., fantasy, erotica, vibrator use), she learned that her body was indeed capable of becoming aroused. The rationale presented to Mona was based on the finding that women's subjective and genital arousal are often desynchronous. By first exciting the mind sexually through fantasy, she could be more likely to tune in to potential signs of arousal in her body during her mindfulness practice. By first exciting her body (with erotica or a vibrator), and then practicing mindfulness immediately afterward, she was able to notice her body's arousal and focus on it. This ultimately enhanced her subjective excitement, for she experienced firsthand that her body was not "broken," and, in fact, was quite responsive. Education about the nature of fantasy emphasized the range of sexual fantasies and challenged Mona's preconception that fantasizing would be synonomous with being unfaithful. She could evoke a sexual fantasy in her mind, and then deliberately focus her attention onto her body, thus enhancing the connection between her mind's and her body's excitement. She struggled coming up with her own fantasy; therefore, she enjoyed reading some of the fantasies provided in books by Nancy Friday (*My Secret Garden, Forbidden Flowers*).

The ultimate result was that Mona had a significant improvement in sexual desire as measured by validated questionnaires and by her own self-report. She began to initiate sexual activity and was more responsive to Harry's advances. By planning sexual activity, she could anticipate sex positively, which improved her sense of self and further enhanced her connection with Harry.

How is mindfulness different from sensate focus? Sensate focus is designed to teach one to increase concentration on the sensual aspects of touching while experiencing relaxation. At this level, mindfulness and sensate focus bear a striking resemblance and one can see aspects of mindfulness (as well as desensitization) in the practice of sensate focus. However, unlike sensate focus, mindfulness is a state of being that can apply to all situations—not only sexual ones. Mindfulness also does not require the presence of a partner, and in fact, in our practice we encourage women to practice mindfulness alone and in nonsexual situations for several weeks before attempting to integrate it into their sexual experiences.

Commentary

After her group sessions Mona became better able to remain focused and present oriented during sexual activity and, in fact, during many nonsexual situations. Changes in her sex life included an increased willingness to accept Harry's invitations to sex, increased arousal during sex, increased ability to tune in to the experienced arousal and thus an increase in sexual desire, reduced distractibility during sex, and reduced frequency of irrational beliefs about sex. Because her tendency to multitask and become distracted was so automatic, the gains she achieved were conditional upon continued mindfulness practice. Clinically we use the analogy that the mind is like a puppy, continually wanting to run this way and that in search of excitement. However, if one wants the mind to stay focused, one needs to guide it back, as if gently tugging on the leash of that puppy. With practice and over time, Mona may become more adept at remaining in the present. However, she will need continued practice in order to realize the full benefits of mindfulness.

CONCLUSION

Overall, we feel the addition of mindfulness to CBT for women with low desire is very helpful. Individual and/or couple sex therapy may then be more targeted to specific needs of the woman and her partner. As East meets West in many other domains of Western medicine, we may increasingly see mindfulness (and other Eastern approaches) being incorporated into the treatment of sexual dysfunction, as well as an increase in empirical efforts to establish its efficacy.

REFERENCES

Beck, A. T. (1993). *Cognitive therapy of depression: A personal reflection.* Aberdeen, Scotland: Scottish Cultural Press.

Brotto, L. A., Basson, R., & Luria, M. (2008). A mindfulness-based group psychoeducational intervention targeting sexual arousal disorder in women. *Journal of Sexual Medicine, 5*, 1646–1659.

Brotto, L. A., Heiman, J. R., Goff, B., Greer, B., Lentz, G. M., Swisher, E., et al. (2008). A psychoeducational intervention for sexual dysfunction in women with gynecologic cancer. *Archives of Sexual Behavior, 37*, 317–329.

Carson, J. W., Carson, K. M., Gil, K. M., & Baucom, D. M. (2004). Mindfulness-based relationship enhancement. *Behavior Therapy, 35*, 471–494.

Ellis, A. (1962). *Reason and emotion in psychotherapy.* New York: Lyle Stuart.

McCabe, M. P. (2001). Evaluation of a cognitive behavior therapy program for people with sexual dysfunction. *Journal of Sex and Marital Therapy, 27,* 259–271.

Trudel, G., Marchand, A., Ravart, M., Aubin, S., Turgeon, L., & Fortier, P. (2001). The effect of a cognitive-behavioral group treatment program on hypoactive sexual desire in women. *Sexual and Relationship Therapy, 16,* 145–164.

if the "spark" was simply gone. Secretly they worried that when the kids were grown, one of them might leave or have an affair. They didn't just miss sex. They missed being "in love." The intoxicating romance. Seeing the glow in each other's eyes. Even the simple comfort of touching and being touched.

My heart ached for them, but I was also hopeful. They'd already made progress in our therapy. We had met eight times and they were fighting less and working together better. They were doing their therapy homework. We knew from the start that they both felt badly about their sexuality and wanted to change. I believed that they could find a way to reach each other's hearts and find renewed pleasure, even joy, in each other's bodies.

**   **   **

What Kit and Jack didn't fully appreciate was how normal their painful difficulties in sustaining an active and intimate sexual life were. Despite our living in a sexually saturated and permissive culture, where virtually every movie theater, magazine, and TV show celebrates copulation, many couples are experiencing a dramatic lessening of sexual libido and activity. In the privacy of their own homes, couples are headed for bed to sleep, not for sex, and often feel either profound shame or blame that ripples through the rest of their relationship. This diminution of desire is true for men and women alike, gay and straight, old and young.

There are many proffered explanations for the large decrease in sexual desire and sexual behavior in long-term couple relationships. One important contribution to low sexual desire for many couples is the complexity and challenge of contemporary life.

In the last 40 years, the majority of couples have become dual-career families, with both working hard outside the home as well as sharing the responsibilities for raising the children and maintaining the home. Couple relationships are no longer as defined by gender roles as they used to be, and the net result is that most couples are trying to negotiate virtually every aspect of their relationship. They are working out how to be wage earners, co-parents, housekeepers, best friends, and lovers. Nonstop negotiations about who will drive Johnny to soccer and who is doing the income tax and whose turn it is to do the food shopping are rarely erotic. Couples are often so intertwined with each other around the business of life that they evolve into a kind of sibling relationship, which may be highly functional but makes sexuality seem almost incestuous. As Esther Perel (2006) emphasizes in her book, *Mating in Captivity*, distance and differentiation are key elements in sustaining erotic energy and mystery.

Another variable is that couples' sexuality is no longer organized by the old, repressive contract that men were entitled to sex in exchange for providing for and protecting women. Today, both men and women want and expect greater intimacy, mutuality, and reciprocity than perhaps ever before in human history. This puts a tremendous pressure on couples to not just "do it" but be "into" doing it. Unfortunately, regardless of gender or sexual orientation, usually one member of the couple wants to be close and intimate before being sexual and one thinks being sexual is a good way of connecting and feeling closer. As with Kit and Jack, the pressure on both members of the couple to feel "in the mood" at the same time and place can be daunting.

Finally, as couples make the transition from being in love to being in life, they have to handle the shift from the intensity of romance to the routines of attachment. Couples often wound each other in the process because they lack the skill to negotiate a mutual understanding about how to fit sexuality and romance into the necessities of life.

I remember treating a couple in their mid-60s and when we were discussing their early marriage the wife burst into tears and told about how she grew up with a lot of sexual energy but, having been given a strict religious upbringing, she had dutifully saved herself for her marriage. Apparently the first few months of the marriage were a sexual Cirque du Soleil for her, but one day she decided to be really bold and surprise her husband when he got home from work. She had put on a slinky black negligee and greeted him at the door with a chilled bottle of champagne and a fluted glass. He opened the door and was startled (and probably anxious, as many men are when confronted with sexually assertive women). He tried to cover his nervousness with a little joke. "What have you've been doing all day, lying around in bed drinking?" he said. The young bride walked out of the room, threw out the champagne and the negligee, and in the ensuing 43 years of marriage never initiated another sexual encounter.

Most couples feel a profound, almost spiritual yearning to be fully known and loved for who they are. However, in the complex business of being a couple, they inevitably bring their flawed and limited humanity. They disappoint each other and cannot meet all of each other's needs. They inadvertently hurt each other, but don't know how to talk that through to resolution. They learn to soldier on, either deflecting conflict or avoiding it, feeling some mix of acceptance and resignation. Rarely can they share their natural sense of disappointment and loss with each other. This separates them. For many, it's like their own experience of being expelled from the Garden of Eden.

SESSION ONE

Kit and Jack didn't come to therapy to work on their sexuality. Most couples come to me for a variety of presenting problems, from affairs, power struggles and conflict, lack of communication, parenting, and money to in-law problems. Many come with one or both members of the couple considering divorce.

I begin all of my couple interviews by focusing on their strengths, what first attracted them to each other, what they like each about other, and what they do best. Most couples soften a little with this emphasis on the positive before we get into their presenting problem. Then, after interviewing them about their difficulties, I ask couples how their issues impact their intimate sexual life. I frequently get a response like Jack's: "What sexual life?" To which Kit responded with an eye roll and a nervous laugh.

I explained:

> "Many couples' struggles have a direct and unfortunately negative impact on their intimate lives. Most couples choose to work on the frustrations and tensions that brought them here first. Everyone tends to assume that if they can be better friends, fight less, and work together better, their sexual intimacy will reignite on its own. Frequently this isn't true. The progress couples make in their relationship often doesn't translate into a better sexual relationship. Issues around sexuality can be difficult to change even when you're feeling closer together. If that happens to you guys, don't panic. I work with a lot of couples around rejuvenating their sex life. Some couples even decide to start there. One couple said that if they could have a good intimate life, their other conflicts and struggles would melt away."

"Well, Dr. Treadway, I think we would have to be feeling a lot closer before dealing with those issues," piped up Kit quickly.

"No problem, Kit. Most couples, particularly most women, want an improvement in the closeness, intimacy, and trust in their relationship before focusing on sex. Sometimes I tease men and say, 'Don't worry, just consider the talking part, foreplay. We'll get there.' "

I was pleased to see that they both smiled, albeit a little shyly. I introduced the issue of sexual intimacy and the notion that it might be necessary to work on it explicitly early in the therapy, but not before they were ready. I usually start by presenting three options for structuring the therapeutic work.

I described the alternatives to Kit and Jack:

> "The first option is putting aside your past hurts, resentments, and blame and focusing on the here and now. The emphasis is on developing new relational skills and ways of communicating, decision making, and nurturing each other.
>
> "The second option, which is especially valuable for couples who have accumulated significant hurt, anger, and mistrust from many painful moments in their relationship, is to put your present relationship on hold, establish a truce, and have zero expectations for improvement. Rather, we would focus on acknowledging your painful history in a safe, compassionate way. You each would have a session or two with your partner and me where both of us would just listen with tenderness and compassion to your accumulated hurts and disappointments. I would help the listening partner put aside defensiveness and self-justification and simply hear and make amends for the harm they've done along the way. Most couples can't talk about their hurts without making it worse. We would work on your being able to open your hearts, apologize, and begin to forgive each other. We would really be working on bringing closure to the marriage you have had, before beginning to work on the relationship you might have.
>
> "The third option is that we would begin with the story of your childhoods and the families you grew up in. For many people, their childhood experiences of love and loss, attachment and isolation, competency and insecurity shape who they grow up to be, what they seek in their intimate relationships, and why their present behavior doesn't work for them. So, we might start

with several sessions exploring those themes before we even get to your wedding day. And, in the meantime, you would go on in your regular way together, even if it's sometimes difficult. For some couples, it helps to have a deeper understanding of their relationship before even beginning to try and change it."

Kit looked overwhelmed. "This is a lot. I have no idea where we should start." Jack nodded.

"Not to worry. There's no right or wrong answer. Couples rarely have the time and the safety to decide together how to work on improving their relationship, how to collaborate on creating a more intimate and satisfying marriage. Let's just pause here."

I gave them each a handout describing the choices. "Take a look at this and let's talk about it."

When they were done reading the choices, I encouraged them to turn toward each other and discuss the possibilities. They didn't know what to say. They had no set speeches of shame or blame, no clarity about right/wrong, good/bad. They were working together on something brand new and potentially exciting for them. They were creating their own therapy model.

Kit was intrigued by the family-of-origin work, because she thought Jack's family had been traumatizing for him. And, in a gender-typical way, Jack wanted to focus on skills going forward, not on rehashing the past. I helped them negotiate, not interrupting each other, showing respect for their different ideas, listening carefully. They were taking ownership of their treatment and learning to work together. They understood that all three elements of their relationship—their past, present, and future—were key to changing their relationship, and that they could not work on everything at once. They would have to learn how to tolerate their unresolved issues, while taking only one step at a time. Therapy had begun.

SESSION SIX

At first they did well. After more discussion, they decided to work on learning new relationship skills. I gave them a talk/listen exercise. They each spend 15 minutes listening carefully and reflecting back, but an important element is that the partners' turns as the talker are separated by at least 24 hours so that the exercise doesn't dissolve into a debate. The emphasis is on each person having a safe place to talk about his or her feelings without rebuttal. I also taught them a nurturing exercise, in which each of them gives the other an explicitly requested, unilateral gift. Enhancing a couple's communication/negotiation skills and capacity for giving and receiving nurture are key to future work on intimacy and sexuality.

Both Jack and Kit had difficulty coming up with gifts they would like to receive from one another. "Listen, you're not alone," I reassured them. "Many couples have difficulty specifying one particular thing. Think in terms of an action, like breakfast in bed or bringing home flowers. Don't ask each other to be kinder or in a better mood. It's got to be something the other can *do*."

They sat quietly for a while and then Kit said, "Well, I would really like it if one night a week we could go to bed a half hour earlier and I could curl up next to Jack and put my head on his chest, and he would read out loud to me from my favorite childhood book, *The Secret Garden*."

Jack smiled tenderly, and said he would be happy to do that. Then, after much hesitation, Jack asked if Kit could draw him a bubble bath and then wash his hair. She reached for his hand and said, "Sure thing, sweetie."

This is going great, I thought to myself.

SESSION EIGHT REVISITED

They continued to make progress, doing better as a parenting team with their kids, not fighting, and doing the talk/listen and "gifting" exercises. But two sessions later, the bottom fell out. Kit arrived in tears and Jack was withdrawn and defensive. The night before, Kit had inadvertently discovered that Jack had been logging on to female-domination pornography sites on their computer. She was devastated.

"I thought things were so much better," she said.

I look at them with compassion and tenderness. I'd hoped they would want to work on their sexuality issues as a result of the positive steps they were making in their relationship. But frequently, couples stumble into their sexual dilemmas like Alice falling down the rabbit hole.

Here they were, hurt, angry, and humiliated. Their lack of frequent sexual engagement didn't mean they had no sexual desires or needs. There's a reason why pornography is the biggest business on the Internet and why women buy vibrators and read romance novels. Jack and Kit had lost the ability to turn toward each other for intimate sexual connection. Instead they had either turned off or turned away.

First, I needed to help Jack move out of shame and defensiveness and help Kit feel less rejected and blamed. I leaned toward her and said gently, "I know it must be horrifying to see some of these aggressive images and to think of Jack being responsive to them."

She nodded, choking back sobs.

I turned toward Jack. "And it's got be incredibly embarrassing for you to have Kit come across this stuff. I mean, there's everything you can imagine on the Internet and a lot of guys—but not just guys—find it easier to get their sexual relief with a click of the mouse than to deal with all the stuff around having a sexual encounter with their partner."

He looked at the floor.

I returned to Kit. "But it's got to be hard for you, when he is kind of making it sound like it's all your fault. I think he's so ashamed that he's lashing out a little. I think he knows perfectly well that the dilemma around maintaining sexual intimacy is a challenge for both of you.

"And you share equal responsibility, Jack. Do you agree?" I was giving him a gentle nudge.

"Yes." He turned to Kit. "And I am really sorry." He started to tear up. "I am so sorry."

She reached out and took his hand. After a long silence, she asked, "Does that stuff I saw mean that's what you want me to do to you?"

"God, no!" he said quickly. "I mean, that's just fantasy, you know. I've never even thought about you and me and—"

Kit started to pull back. We were getting ahead of ourselves.

"Listen, you two, there's a lot to talk about here. Almost everybody has powerful erotic fantasies, and many couples never share them with each other. Just because something's a turn-on in someone's mind doesn't mean that they want to act it out. Kit, what could Jack do that would help repair things?"

"Well, Dr. Treadway, I . . . "

"Speak to him."

"I'd like it if you didn't go on those Internet sites anymore secretly."

"I can do that," Jack replied.

"Good. That's a start. You have been going great in our work together. Maybe it's time to open up the conversation about your intimate life and explore how to rejuvenate your sexual intimacy. Would you be willing to do a simple exercise to kind of get started?"

"Depends on what it is," Jack said, warily.

"We'll try it and if it's too uncomfortable for either of you, we'll stop, okay?"

They both nodded.

"Kit, turn on the sofa so your back is to Jack, and Jack, you slide toward her so that you can comfortably massage her shoulders. Is that okay with you, Kit?"

"I guess."

"So we'll give it a try, and in a few moments we'll change positions and you'll give him a massage. Could you both close your eyes? And while this gentle massage is happening, I want each of you to just feel whatever feelings you have."

Jack began to massage Kit's shoulders while I talked to them. "Each of you may be experiencing a whole host of emotions, starting with how contrived and silly this exercise feels … "

Jack chuckled.

"But also, Kit, you may be feeling wary and distrustful, ambivalent about whether you even want Jack to be touching you right now. Or you may feel self-conscious with me being here and even frustrated that it's hard to relax and enjoy yourself. While Jack, you might feel on the spot and not sure how to give a comforting massage or whether Kit's just going through the motions to be a good sport in therapy. You may be worried about what Kit's feeling. I'd like both of you to experience this touch while feeling whatever emotions are going on and try not to worry about what you think you should be feeling.

"Now let's pause before we switch and hear some of your feelings."

"That felt pretty gimmicky and I was pretty confident she was tense about it."

"That's fine, Jack. And how about for you, Kit?"

"It made me sad. We don't ever touch each other that way anymore. To be honest, I'd prefer for us to be able to do this at home and not have to be in your office. But actually, it felt kind of good," she said, softly.

"Well, the whole idea behind this exercise is that all couples develop a mixed up mess of feelings toward each other as they make their way through life. In one way or another, you've hurt each other a lot through the years, and this episode with the Internet porn is only one of many things that have been difficult.

"For couples to be truly intimate in the bedroom, you have to be comfortable with your own sad/mad/bad feelings that have accumulated. It is truly liberating when you can bring all of yourselves, including your bad feelings, to each other in the bedroom without shame, blame, and fear. And still make love. You can discover that you have these hurt, resistant, even angry emotions and let it all be part of your intimate touch. Instead of what most couples do, which is try to sweep it under the rug in order to be sexual, an approach that makes for lumpy rugs and lousy sex."

The session was very painful but very intimate, and it ended with their feeling closer. The core reason why couples withdraw from sexuality is that true intimacy is very hard. The touching exercise introduced the idea that Kit and Jack could have gentle touch while still acknowledging difficult feelings. Most people think intimacy is supposed to be a feel-good experience, a Hallmark card event. Often, it hurts. Being able to share the hurts allows couples to be fully present to each other and to learn how to make love with each other's whole selves.

SESSION TEN

"We're ready for the experiments, Dr. Treadway," says Kit with a giggle and a shy smile at Jack.

They're sitting on the sofa, holding hands. Last session, we reviewed their sexual history and considered whether there were any medical, psychopharmacological, or trauma-based reasons for their pattern of sexual avoidance. They had had garden-variety difficulties: too little time, too high expectations, kids underfoot, too much fighting, and so on. We agreed that instead of dealing with their past and their history of hurts and disappointments about their sexual life, they would try different approaches. They were ready to risk a few trial-and-error experiments, but I cautioned them first.

"Just as in the beginning, when you two negotiated and designed your own therapeutic approach, it will be very important for you to explore together what might be the best way to start working on your sexual intimacy. The main thing you have to accept, though, is that whatever we choose it will involve work, scheduling, organizing. And learning to be comfortable with ambivalent, resistant, anxious, discouraged, and even angry feelings. Most people yearn for easy spontaneity and mutual desire and responsiveness. They just want to flow together the way Fred Astaire and Ginger Rogers danced. They want sex to be relaxed, romantic, even playful. So it's hard to accept how hard you actually have to work at it.

"Let me give you a menu of possibilities for getting started. Would that be okay?"

They nod, with slightly anxious smiles.

"Here are four choices and either of you may have your own proposals as to how to begin. The first is simply talking and each of you sharing your own unfolding story as a young child, sharing your private experiences about sexuality and gender as you developed. You might talk about your first awareness of being a boy or a girl, how affection and sexuality were expressed between your parents, your earliest sexual feelings, imagery, touch, experience of puberty, first crush, first kiss, and so forth. Exploring all the tender, shy vulnerability that is still deep within each of you. I have a questionnaire that you can use at home or we could even do it here, if you prefer."

I could tell that Kit liked this idea but I kept going.

"Second, since you did so well with the giving and receiving exercise, you could set aside a time each week when one of you would give and receive sexual pleasuring; or, if you're not ready for receiving that, simply giving and receiving sensual massage. It will help you guide each other. Ironically, both men and women often have difficulty receiving pleasure without reciprocity, so it's a huge step forward as part of your sexual repertoires to simply learn to take turns.

"Third, very few couples are comfortable really being seductive with each other, nor do they know how to turn their partner down lovingly and affirmingly when they aren't feeling responsive. Some of the couples in my practice learn to lighten up by role playing. One night one member of the couple has the challenge of being seductive, while knowing that their partner has the challenge of declining the seduction in a loving, appreciative way.

"Finally, some couples benefit from deciding that intercourse and orgasm are off limits. They just practice the adolescent joys of making out with clothes on, but not in the bedroom. Experimenting with being sexual in a different place—the kitchen, the car, or even between floors in an elevator. This allows for playful flirtation without performance pressure. Actually, my wife and I tried this out in the high school parking lot once after going to a movie. Believe it or not, we got busted! A cop banged on the car window and flashed his flashlight on us. He was young enough to be our son. There we were, me with my bald pate and my wife with her silver hair. He turned red."

Kit and Jack chuckled. I often throw something in the mix about the vagaries and comedy of my own sexual history as a way of defusing the tension and creating a little humor around the issue.

"So that's a lot to start with and you may have entirely different ways to engage each other. What do you think?"

Naturally, Kit and Jack chose differently. She liked the idea of talking about their childhood experiences and he was responsive to taking turns giving pleasure. It didn't matter that they disagreed. They could negotiate and experiment. They could even flip a coin.

My job was to create a safe, nurturing environment when they could open to each other. Now it was their time to write their own love song, dance to their own music.

CONCLUSION

Over the ensuing five sessions, Kit and Jack tried a variety of experiments and exercises with some pleasant surprises and some duds. We had a very sweet session about their childhood sexuality, and the power of Jack's responsiveness to female domination seemed directly linked to his highly critical and dominating mother, who he both rebelled against and desperately wanted to please. Jack was very open and vulnerable and Kit was able to be empathic and compassionate about how these painful issues could be expressed through sexual desires, but she still didn't want him to turn away from her and toward the Internet. Jack readily agreed to this but I worried aloud whether he would be able to stick to it or just go underground again. The taking turns strategy actually increased their frequency of sexual engagement, which did help Jack feel less bad about his sexual drive and Kit feel less pressure to "be in the mood" every time. They also tried the seduction/rejection game and found it too silly and contrived. But mostly what happened was that they learned to talk with each other, nurture each other, and accept the inevitable compromises in their sexual relationship with grace and tenderness. Jack and Kit found their own rhythm as they rediscovered each other, the man and woman they had become, and learned to truly make love with each other.

COMMENTARY

In telling their story, I've tried to show the core of what I do to help couples work with their struggles around sexual incompatibility, lack of desire, and intimacy. Of course, not all stories work out so well. Each couple has to find their own gentle balance between resignation and acceptance, daring to try changing, yet embracing each other as they are.

Clearly therapists, myself included, have to consider many elements in working with couples who have low sexual desire. Age, biological and medical factors, gender differences, relationship issues, and trauma history may all be significant variables.

There were several key ingredients in my work with Kit and Jack; most of these are obvious and much practiced by many of my colleagues who work with these difficult issues.

1. Building a safe and nurturing therapeutic environment.
2. Helping the couple design their own therapeutic protocol of either going forward or dealing with past, even the family of origin, while tolerating the limitations of unresolved and difficult issues that are deferred by their choice.
3. Normalizing their difficulties and helping them feel less bad about themselves as a couple.
4. Helping them learn how to communicate difficult feelings to each other and how to give and receive nurturance well.

5. Helping them accept the necessity of prioritizing and scheduling to make time for each other.
6. Teaching them how to be emotionally open with each other, including discussing their hurt/anger/mistrust, while also enjoying relaxed sensuality and touch.
7. Helping them reduce their performance anxiety and expectations. I encourage couples to accept a modicum of mediocre, ho-hum sexuality instead of always expecting fireworks. This increases the chance that the "magic" will happen some of the time.
8. Encouraging them to choose their own therapeutic homework and creative experiments.

The heart of the work with all couples lies in helping them become more comfortable with their discomforts and differences and able to share their feelings without shame or shoulds, and hear each other's feelings without taking them too personally. Both members of every couple need to learn how to be carefully true to themselves while in the presence of the other, to apologize and forgive, and to accept the flaws of each other's shared humanity—and, finally, to adopt the Serenity Prayer (accepting the things they cannot change and having the courage to change the things they can) as a way of life.

Then they can learn a new dance.

BIBLIOGRAPHY

Bischoff, R. J., McKeel, A. J., Moon, S. M., & Sprenkle, D. H. (1996). Therapist-conducted consultation: Using clients as consultants to their own therapy. *Journal of Marital and Family Therapy, 22*(3), 359–379

Gottman, J. M. (1999). *The marriage clinic: A scientifically-based marital therapy*. New York: Norton.

Gurman, A. S., & Jacobson, N. S. (2002). *Clinical handbook of couples therapy* (3rd ed.). New York: Guilford Press.

Leiblum, S. R., & Rosen, R. C. (Eds.). (2000). *Principles and practice of sex therapy*. New York: Guilford Press.

McCarthy, B. (2004). *Rekindling desire: A step-by-step program to help low-sex and no-sex marriages*. New York: Brunner-Routledge.

Mellody, P., & Freundlich, L. S. (2003). *The intimacy factor: The ground rules for overcoming the obstacles to truth, respect, and lasting love*, San Francisco: HarperCollins.

Perel, E. (2006). *Mating in captivity: Unblocking erotic intelligence.* New York: HarperCollins.

Schnarch, D. (1997). *Passionate marriage: Sex, love and intimacy in emotionally committed relationships.* New York: Norton.

Stuart, R. B. (2003). *Helping couples change: A social learning approach to marital therapy.* New York: Guilford Press.

Treadway, D. (1994, March/April). In a world of their own. *Family Therapy Networker,* 32–39.

Chapter 11

Treatment of Low Sexual Desire in the Context of Comorbid Individual and Relationship Dysfunction

Douglas K. Snyder

In this chapter, Douglas K. Snyder highlights the relationship dynamics that so critically contribute to, and often exacerbate, sexual desire complaints. While acknowledging the value of psychological exploration of each partner's psychodynamic and developmental issues that may be thwarting sexual desire, Snyder suggests a more flexible approach—one in which a collaborative alliance between the partners is first achieved and the major couple conflicts are addressed before dealing with the sexual difficulties. He recommends a "pluralistic affective reconstructive approach", wherein each partner becomes more aware of, and empathic to the other's emotional needs and struggles, so that better communication and greater receptivity—both emotional and sexual—can be achieved.

Through the use of sample dialogue, Snyder illustrates how gently challenging and encouraging couples to reconsider how they speak to, and think about, each other paves the way for more effective communication and empathic responding. While an improvement in marital harmony and appreciation is achieved, the change in sexual desire is less dramatic. And, in truth, this is usually the outcome in most cases involving a sexual desire discrepancy—actual increases in sexual frequency are often modest despite greatly enhanced couple satisfaction.

Douglas K. Snyder, PhD, is Professor and Director of Clinical Training in the Department of Psychology at Texas A&M University in College Station, Texas. In addition to being a preeminent couple therapist, he (along with his two colleagues, Donald Baucom and Kristina Gordon) is the author of a popular book on dealing with the aftermath of an affair entitled *Getting Past the Affair: A Program to Help You Cope, Heal, and Move On—Together or Apart.*

Both clinical case illustrations and empirical literature document the multifaceted structure of low sexual desire, both in terms of subjective phenomenology and underlying etiologies. From a phenomenological perspective—in addition to prevalent or generalized lack of subjective feelings of desire—individuals may report low levels of sexual responsiveness in the presence of appropriate stimulation or approaches by an intimate partner, limited mental imagery related to sexual interactions, infrequent or negative sexual thoughts, or absence of sexual drive or energy not consistent with vigor in other individual or interpersonal domains. Etiologically, the literature cites similarly diverse and sometimes interacting causes potentially contributing to low sexual desire—including biological, psychological, interpersonal, and broader systemic factors.

This chapter describes a framework for conceptualizing low sexual desire and organizing therapeutic interventions from diverse theoretical perspectives with couples distinguished by comorbid individual and relationship dysfunction. In this context, "individual dysfunction" refers to significant emotional or behavioral disorders extending beyond low sexual desire to include substantial affective or cognitive dysfunction and/or personality disturbance as defined by diagnostic criteria enumerated in the *Diagnostic and Statistical Manual of Mental Disorders* (DSM-IV-TR; American Psychiatric Association, 2000). Similarly, "relationship dysfunction" refers to relational difficulties extending beyond partners' discrepant levels of sexual desire to include high levels of conflict, low levels of emotional or physical intimacy outside the sexual domain, inadequate communication skills involving either decision making or emotional expressiveness, or notable deficits in other domains related to developing and maintaining interpersonal closeness. Adopting this emphasis does not presume that cases of low sexual desire necessarily or even predominantly include significant individual or relationship dysfunction. Rather, this chapter's focus evolves from the author's specialty clinical practice emphasizing almost exclusively couple-based interventions with complex cases in which typically one or both partners have already been diagnosed with individual psychopathology comorbid with presenting problems of significant couple distress.

EMPIRICAL AND THEORETICAL RATIONALE

Findings Regarding Comorbidity

The conceptual framework advocated here derives in part from the broader empirical literature documenting that relationship difficulties often co-occur with significant emotional, behavioral, and physical health problems in one or both partners (see Snyder & Whisman, 2003, for detailed descriptions of couple-based interventions for cases of coexisting mental and relationship disorders). For example, in comparison to nondistressed individuals, maritally distressed individuals are three times more likely to have a mood disorder, 2.5 times more likely to have an anxiety disorder, and two times more likely to have a substance use disorder (Whisman, 2006). Moreover, findings indicate that the presence of mental health problems is associated with greater marital distress, above and beyond general distress in other close relationships. Evidence also indicates that both physical health and adjustment to physical health problems are positively associated with relationship quality. For example, in a study on psychological adjustment of adults with cancer, Rodrigue and Park (1996) found that people with high relationship distress reported more depression and anxiety, a less positive health care orientation, and more illness-induced family difficulties. The preponderance of empirical evidence indicates that relationship functioning, particularly negative communication, has direct effects on cardiovascular, endocrine, immune, neurosensory, and other physiological systems that, in turn, affect health (Kiecolt-Glaser & Newton, 2001). Hence, to the extent that sexual desire is susceptible to adverse influences of mood disorders, substance use, and general health, one could anticipate sexual difficulties generally, and low sexual desire specifically, to be linked to generalized relationship distress.

Indeed, more than 30 years of research has demonstrated disproportionately higher incidence of difficulties in couples' sexual relationships in the presence of more generalized couple distress. For example, in a mixed group of 2,140 individuals from combined representative community and clinical samples, Snyder and Whisman (2004) determined that individuals reporting moderate or high global relationship distress on a multidimensional measure of relationship functioning (the Marital Satisfaction Inventory—Revised (MSI-R; Snyder, 1997) were 6.2 times more likely to report moderate or extensive dissatisfaction with their sexual relationship than individuals reporting only low levels of general couple distress. On the basis of findings from this same measure, Berg and Snyder (1981) outlined two situations in which the clinician would be prudent to defer brief directive sex therapy in favor of more extensive marital therapy: (1) when levels of global couple distress exceed moderate proportions, or (2) when one or both partners report primary distress around nonsexual aspects of their relationship such as communication or emotional intimacy.

An Informed Pluralistic Approach to Couple Therapy

Couple therapists confront a tremendous diversity of presenting issues, marital and family structures, individual dynamics and psychopathology, and psychosocial stressors characterizing couples in distress. Because the functional sources of couples' distress vary so dramatically, the critical mediators or mechanisms of change should also be expected to vary—as should the therapeutic strategies intended to facilitate positive change. Couples with comorbid individual and relationship dysfunctions will benefit most from a treatment strategy drawing from both conceptual and technical innovations from diverse theoretical models relevant to different components of a couple's struggles. Snyder (1999) advocated a pluralistic approach to couple therapy conceptualizing therapeutic tasks as progressing sequentially along a hierarchy comprising six levels of intervention, from the most fundamental interventions promoting a collaborative alliance to more challenging interventions addressing developmental sources of relationship distress. Because couple therapy often proceeds in nonlinear fashion, the model depicts flexibility in returning to earlier therapeutic tasks as dictated by individual or relationship difficulties (see Figure 11.1). Pluralism recognizes the validity of multiple systems of epistemology, theory, and practice and draws on these as intact units in an integrative manner by adhering to an explicit and orderly model of treatment selection.

As depicted in Figure 11.1, the most fundamental step in couple therapy involves developing a collaborative alliance between partners and between each partner and the therapist by establishing an atmosphere of therapist competence as well as therapeutic safety around

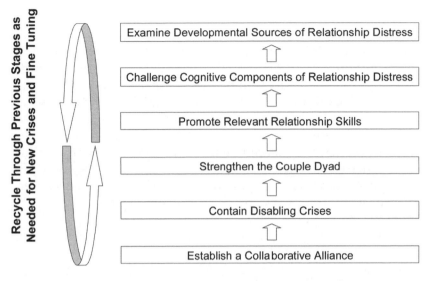

Primary Therapeutic Task

FIGURE 11.1. A sequential, pluralistic approach to couple therapy. The model depicts progression from (1) lower-order interventions aimed at establishing a collaborative alliance and crisis containment, through (2) positive-exchange and skills-building techniques, to (3) higher-order interventions targeting cognitive and developmental sources of relationship distress. Couple therapy may include recycling through earlier stages as required by emergent crises or erosion of individual or relationship skills.

issues of confidentiality and verbal or physical aggression. Subsequent interventions may need to target disabling relationship crises such as substance use, psychopathology, illness or death of a family member, infidelity, or similar concerns that—until resolved—preclude development of new relationship skills and progress toward emotional intimacy. Because some couples initially present with overwhelming negativity, the therapist may need to instigate behavior change directly before assisting the couple to develop behavior-exchange and communication skills of their own. Along with promoting general relationship skills, the couple therapist may need to assist partners in acquiring a prerequisite knowledge base and competence in specific domains such as parenting, finances, or time management.

A common impediment to behavior change involves misconceptions and other interpretive errors that individuals may have regarding both their own and their partner's behavior; such cognitive influences are particularly relevant to persons' views of their own and their partner's sexuality. Interventions targeting partners' relationship beliefs, expectancies, and attributions aim to eliminate or restructure cognitive processes interfering with behavior change efforts. However, not all psychological processes relevant to couples' interactions—sexual or otherwise—lend themselves to traditional cognitive interventions. Of particular importance are partners' developmental relationship experiences resulting in enduring interpersonal vulnerabilities and related defensive strategies interfering with emotional or sexual intimacy, many of which operate beyond partners' conscious awareness. Hence, when couple distress persists despite system-restructuring, skills-building, and cognitive interventions, then interpretation of maladaptive relationship patterns evolving from developmental processes comprises an essential treatment component (Snyder & Mitchell, 2008).

With respect to the treatment of low sexual desire, this pluralistic approach presumes that couples will vary in the extent to which they require interventions at any level of the treatment hierarchy but also presumes that higher-order interventions (e.g., cognitive or insight-oriented techniques targeting intrapersonal processes) would ordinarily not be implemented unless lower-order interventions (e.g., crisis intervention, relationship strengthening, or skills-building techniques targeting interpersonal processes) had already proven insufficient.

The following case illustrates implementation of this pluralistic approach in treating low sexual desire in a woman with comorbid dysthymia and a prior history of vaginismus, compounded by significant marital difficulties and enduring emotional issues in both partners rooted in early developmental experiences.

CASE EXAMPLE: DON AND CAROL

Presenting Problems

Don and Carol were referred for couple therapy by Carol's primary physician. The couple presented with extensive difficulties in their sexual relationship stemming primarily from Carol's lack of interest in sexual relations. Don preferred intercourse at least once or twice weekly, whereas Carol was content with sexual relations once a month or less. With the exception of their sexual relationship, both partners described their marriage as "a good friendship," although

Carol was somewhat more willing than Don to acknowledge pervasive difficulties in their communication patterns. Among other concerns, she referred to Don's emotional aloofness—a trait that at times also characterized his approach to lovemaking.

The couple had been married 3.5 years and had not been sexually intimate prior to marriage. Carol stated that during latter stages of their courtship, they had become more physically intimate but stopped short of intercourse. Don had viewed these exchanges positively, but Carol disclosed that she had felt emotionally distressed and guilty at the same time she had felt physically aroused. Their first attempt at intercourse after marriage had been painful, which Carol attributed to their both having been sexually inexperienced. Sexual relations continued to be difficult and painful for Carol for months after their marriage. Carol was diagnosed with vaginismus and had been given a set of dilators to use, but stated that she had little motivation to use these, as reflected in her consistent "forgetting" to proceed through the dilation exercises. Only when the urge to have children impelled her to address this problem directly did Carol initiate and maintain vaginal dilation exercises and eventually overcome this difficulty.

Following the birth of their daughter 2 years into their marriage, Carol developed significant and enduring clinical depression. Her dysthymia was initially attributed to postpartum depression and treated with sertraline hydrochloride; although Carol's low sexual desire predated her dysthymia and initial antidepressant medications, pharmacotherapy was altered to bupropion to minimize adverse libidinal side effects. Although Carol's depression lifted somewhat, her low sexual desire persisted. Her physician suggested to Carol that she and Don would likely benefit from couple therapy targeting significant marital difficulties that Carol had disclosed. Don acknowledged ambivalence about this assessment, and suggested that Carol's sexual difficulties may relate more directly to her upbringing, which included strong negative attitudes toward sexuality.

Diagnostic Assessment

The clinical interview revealed that both partners had been reared in highly conservative religious environments that espoused a hierarchical structure for spousal roles and restrictive if not negative views of sexuality. Carol was the oldest of eight children, had extensive responsibilities in caring for her younger siblings as a teenager, and had vowed not to replicate her mother's role of submission to an autocratic husband. Indeed, in Don she had chosen someone who was gentle mannered but also somewhat passive and emotionally aloof. Don was the second of six children and had an older sister who had died in adolescence. He had learned to escape his mother's depression and his father's frequent criticisms by retreating to his bedroom for extended periods throughout his adolescence—a pattern of avoidance he replicated in his marriage. Both partners had been in individual therapy as undergraduates—Carol to address conflicts with her father, in a process she found only modestly helpful, and Don for assistance with his own depression.

Both Don and Carol were graduate teaching assistants in different programs at a local university. Each felt overwhelmed by their respective responsibilities, with Carol reporting inadequate time for her studies because of child-care responsibilities at home, and Don alluding to academic requirements that at times seemed beyond his ability. They each cited little leisure time together at home as a concern. Don attributed this to Carol's lack of enthusiasm for computer games he enjoyed, whereas Carol ascribed their lack of interaction to Don's persistent retreat into solitary pursuits.

Both partners completed the MSI-R (Snyder, 1997), a multidimensional measure of relationship functioning composed of 150 true–false items, with strong psychometric underpinnings and empirical relation to treatment outcome (Snyder et al., 2004). The MSI-R includes two validity scales, a measure of global relationship distress, and 10 additional scales assessing satisfaction with the couple's sexual relationship, affective and problem-solving communication, aggression, leisure time together, finances, and interactions regarding children—in addition to measures of role attitudes and family-of-origin distress. Sample items assessing global distress include "Our relationship has been disappointing in several ways" and "At times I have very much wanted to leave my partner." Sample items assessing satisfaction with the sexual relationship include "My partner sometimes shows too little enthusiasm for sex" and "My partner has too little regard sometimes for my sexual satisfaction." Partners' raw scores on each scale, reflecting the number of items answered in the scored (distressed) direction, are converted to normalized T-scores with a mean of 50 and standard deviation of 10. In most domains (including Global Distress and Sexual Dissatisfaction), scores of 50–60T suggest moderate levels of distress, whereas scores $\geq 61T$ reflect more extensive distress in that domain.

In many respects Carol and Don described their marriage in similar terms on the MSI-R, citing extensive difficulties in their sexual relationship as their primary concern, but also citing moderate concerns with shared leisure time together and overall relationship distress (see Figure 11.2). In comparison to Don, Carol reported more deficits in their communication—particularly involving emotional expressiveness and understanding—as well as more extensive conflicts regarding her family of origin. Interpretive feedback to the couple regarding their MSI-R profiles affirmed their primary concerns about their sexual relationship but also afforded the therapist opportunity to cite communication difficulties and deficits in both emotional and behavioral intimacy as potential contributing causes to Carol's low sexual desire—feedback aimed at encouraging Don to reframe Carol's sexual responsiveness within a broader systemic perspective.

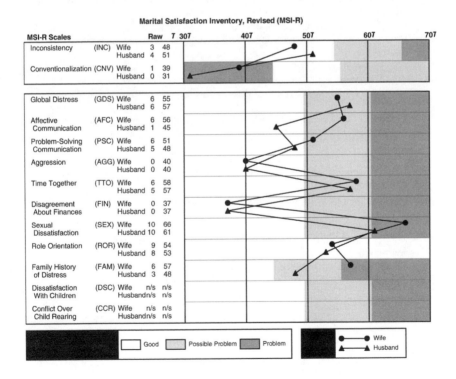

FIGURE 11.2. MSI-R profiles for Don and Carol at initial assessment.

Treatment Course

Treatment of Carol and Don progressed through six levels of intervention, consistent with the hierarchical pluralistic approach described earlier. Exemplars of interventions at each level are provided in Table 11.1, and they are described in greater detail below.

Initial Interventions

After offering a clinical formulation to the couple emphasizing likely contributions to Carol's low sexual desire from multiple sources including biological, psychological, relational, and broader sys-

TABLE 11.1. Interventions with Don and Carol Using a Hierarchical Pluralistic Approach

Level 6—Examine developmental sources of relationship distress.
- Explore and resolve Don's enduring fears of inadequacy contributing to avoidance behaviors.
- Explore and resolve Carol's enduring conflicts around femininity (extending beyond sexuality) contributing to ineffective patterns of engaging and responding to Don.

Level 5—Challenge cognitive components of relationship distress.
- Challenge Don's cognitive distortions and overgeneralization of Carol's complaints.
- Challenge Carol's negative views of sexuality and promote expanded acceptance and expression of sexual feelings.

Level 4—Promote relevant relationship skills.
- Challenge couple's demand → withdraw pattern and promote improved decision-making skills.
- Promote Don's emotional expressiveness skills.

Level 3—Strengthen the couple dyad.
- Modify couple's interactions around sexual requests contributing to verbal aggression.
- Challenge Don's avoidance patterns and promote more active role as a husband and father.

Level 2—Contain disabling crises.
- Address individual and relationship factors contributing to Carol's depression.

Level 1—Establish a collaborative alliance.
- Frame couple's complaint of low sexual desire from a systemic perspective with multiple contributing factors.
- Conduct relevant clinical assessment and develop a shared formulation.

temic considerations, initial interventions targeted those factors most directly related to Carol's overall levels of energy. While allowing that Don was not *responsible* for Carol's low sexual desire, he was encouraged to be *responsive* to her low desire by intervening where possible in processes that might be contributing to her generalized fatigue. Specifically, the therapist encouraged Don to consider a more egalitarian approach to spousal roles and to assist with housework and parenting responsibilities he had previously ascribed primarily to Carol. He was only modestly equipped for these, given the absence of such male role models in his family of origin but was moderately receptive toward specific directives offered by his male therapist, whom he generally trusted as advocating a healthier sexual relationship. In turn, Carol benefitted from explicit directives from the therapist to relax the stringent criteria she held regarding housework and parenting—not only on Don's behalf, but on her own as well. With Don's support, she undertook modest self-care initiatives to attend more faithfully to her need for sleep, exercise, and occasional interactions with women friends.

The couple described a classic pattern of avoiding sexual approaches or discussion of their sexual relationship. Don feared Carol's rejection of his sexual overtures and tended to brood privately about their low rate of sexual exchanges. He stayed up late at night after Carol had gone to bed to avoid the impulse to approach her sexually, but then slept late during the morning, which in turn exacerbated Carol's resentment about his lack of assistance with child care. Their sexual repertoire was also highly constricted in terms of both content and timing of sexual exchanges. With encouragement, Don became more willing to approach Carol sexually and to tolerate occasional rejection of his overtures. Carol learned to communicate more clearly when she did not want sexual exchanges, without an aggressive style she had previously used as a means to cover her feelings of guilt or embarrassment. She also became receptive to suggesting sexual relations at times during the day when she had higher energy, and to tolerate doing so even when housework remained undone. Don was receptive to information about gender differences in arousal patterns and became somewhat more effective in promoting a sexually conducive atmosphere and stimulating Carol before attempting intercourse. Concurrent with his progress in this regard, Carol found it easier to become sexually aroused, although she remained resistant to exploring different ways of satisfying Don sexually. However, over several weeks, resentments about their discrepant desires for sexual intercourse diminished, and their frequency of sexual exchanges showed a modest increase.

Intermediate Interventions

Initial directives aimed specifically at altering structural elements of the couple's relationship to promote sharing of household responsibilities, reduce Carol's generalized fatigue, and increase the range of potential sexual exchanges produced noticeable but limited improvements in the couple's sexual relationship. Constraining further gains were more enduring relationship difficulties in promoting intimacy and negotiating change around allocation of household tasks. Carol and Don demonstrated a prototypical demand → withdraw pattern of communication in which Don's passive retreat and Carol's entreaties for assistance progressively escalated. Similar to Don's style for dealing with their sexual relationship, Carol brooded about Don's passivity until her levels of frustration mounted and her requests assumed an intense and frequently critical tone. Therapeutic interventions emphasized her adopting an assertive but more regulated approach to seeking Don's engagement. Don benefitted from interventions that helped him not to generalize Carol's complaints as indictments of his character or indications of his inadequacy—particularly once Carol learned to link her requests for assistance to the subsequent potential for more shared leisure time together, which sometimes culminated in sexual intimacy. Don struggled with a limited view of emotional or behavioral intimacy. He had difficulty labeling or describing his own feelings and even greater limitations in recognizing or responding to Carol's. Retreat was his preferred response, and this behavioral tendency needed to be addressed in therapy directly.

THERAPIST: So what's it like when Carol lets you know she's frustrated with you?

DON: I don't like it.

THERAPIST: And then what?

DON: I just tune her out.

THERAPIST: And how does that work?

DON: (*after a pause*) Not too well, I guess. I mean, I guess it helps me not to think about what she's saying. But she just gets madder and madder with me—and soon we're either yelling at each other or I just leave.

THERAPIST: Would you be willing to tolerate her being frustrated with you?

DON: I don't like it.

THERAPIST: No, but would you be willing to tolerate it? What do you think would eventually happen?

DON: Well, I guess I could survive it, if that's what you mean—but I think I'd end up feeling worse about myself.

THERAPIST: Could you share that with Carol? Could you say something like, "Look—when you start telling me how I'm never helpful and not a responsible husband or father, I end up feeling even worse and want to pull back even further"?

DON: How would that help?

THERAPIST: Well, then you could offer her an alternative—something like "It would help if you could just let me know what you need in this moment, and then maybe suggest a time window for getting it done instead of my feeling like you're ordering me about like a little boy."

DON: I don't know how she'd like that.

THERAPIST: Try checking it out with Carol.

DON: Okay—so, Carol, how would you like that?

CAROL: Well, if it were said respectfully, I could handle that. I don't mean to order you about, Don. I just get frustrated and feel abandoned by you—and then I take it out on you sometimes by the things I say. I can try to do better at that if you'll just talk with me instead of going into your shell.

Final Interventions

Gradually the couple's overall relationship improved, and their frequency of sexual interactions increased. At the same time, the partners' levels of sexual desire remained discrepant and, compared to modal couples in their age group and circumstances, their frequency of sexual exchanges was relatively low. Once Carol experienced Don's willingness to examine his own contributions to their marriage and she no longer anticipated that he held her singularly responsible for the quality of their sexual relationship, she became more willing to examine in therapy her enduring conflicts around her own sexuality. Although Carol could have explored such conflicts in individual therapy, there were distinct advantages to her doing so within conjoint therapy involving Don's participation. Specifically, as participant-observers in their partner's work on developmental issues, individuals frequently come to understand their partner's behaviors in a more accepting or benign manner—attributing damaging exchanges to the culmination of acquired interpersonal dispositions rather than to explicit motives to be hurtful. This new understanding often facilitates in-session exchanges challenging existing relationship schemas, reducing defensive behaviors, and promoting empathic and mutually supportive interactions (Snyder, 1999; Snyder & Mitchell, 2008).

In this case, Carol began to disclose deeply conflicted feelings about her sexuality once Don stopped blaming her for all the difficulties in their sexual relationship. As she expressed these conflicts in a more openly painful manner, he relinquished his own defensiveness and offered her considerable understanding. More important, his empathic response to Carol's conflicted sexuality extended outside of the treatment sessions to include more supportive responses at home. That is, Don became better able to temper his frustrations over their low sexual activity with softened expressions of disappointment integrated with statements of understanding. Over time this led to cycles of sexual avoidance that were less frequent, shorter in duration, and characterized by considerably less intense exchanges of negative feelings. Therapeutic interventions characteristic of exploring developmental components of low sexual desire are exemplified in the following exchange.

CAROL: I recognized this past week that I was still pulling away from Don when he approached me sexually, even when other parts of our marriage had been going better.

THERAPIST: And what additional thoughts or feelings did you have about that?

CAROL: I don't know—confusion, maybe. Sadness.

THERAPIST: Sadness?

CAROL: Yeah, because that's really not how I want it to be for us. I mean, I think my parents' marriage was pretty empty emotionally, and I wanted more for Don and me.

THERAPIST: More emotional connection.

CAROL: Yes.

THERAPIST: More passion?

CAROL: Well, yes—I guess. I mean, when I was growing up and reading those cheap romance novels, I actually thought that would be pretty neat.

THERAPIST: And now?

CAROL: (*smiling*) I still think it would be neat.

THERAPIST: So what gets in the way?

CAROL: (*after a long pause*) I don't know. I mean, I wanted so much not to be like my mother.

THERAPIST: In what ways?

CAROL: You know—submissive, unemotional, inert.

THERAPIST: And in what ways do you think you may have wanted to be *like* your mom?

CAROL: What do you mean?

THERAPIST: Well, she wasn't all bad, was she? What did you admire about her? What pieces of her might you have wanted to take inside of you for yourself?

CAROL: (*another pause*) I admired her commitment—to her marriage, and to the church. I didn't always agree with the substance of those commitments, but I admired that she followed through with what she believed in.

THERAPIST: You admired her perseverance and also her fidelity.

CAROL: Yes, I did.

THERAPIST: What about her spontaneity, or her emotional expressiveness?

CAROL: Well, those didn't exactly go with the other, right? I mean, to be committed and spontaneous seems contradictory.

THERAPIST: I'm wondering if that belief leads to the contradiction you feel internally.

CAROL: What do you mean?

THERAPIST: Well, I'm struck by your admiration of your mom's commitment. But you clearly didn't admire her submissiveness or the emotional vacuum of your parents' marriage. You've talked before about your lingering resentments about your father's bullying her and later his domineering style with you. But it also seems that his intensity, in his better moments, had an inner strength and a kind of passion about life—even if that was expressed primarily in his work and less about his family. Overtly, you identify more closely with your mom mostly in terms of her values—but on another level there are important parts of her you reject.

CAROL: Yes ...

THERAPIST: And overtly you reject identifying with your father, even though in terms of your own emotional reactivity you're probably not entirely unlike him.

CAROL: And that bothers me.

THERAPIST: I'm wondering if you could find ways of taking the healthier parts of each of them and putting them together in ways that work better for you.

CAROL: How?

THERAPIST: Well, how do you think that might look in terms of your sexual relationship?

CAROL: I don't know.

THERAPIST: (after waiting) Give it a shot.

CAROL: (after a long pause) Well, I guess sometimes it would mean responding to Don's wishes to have sex without my viewing it as my being submissive.

THERAPIST: Giving, rather than giving in ...

CAROL: Exactly ... (another pause) ... and I guess I could resist triggering my automatic "off" switch whenever thinking about sex, and leave it on.

DON: (interrupting) Or at least in "neutral" mode.

THERAPIST: (to Carol) That's harder for you.

CAROL: It is so hard for me. We were so ingrained to view sex as wrong—especially before marriage—but it never became okay or wonderful for me in its own right, even after marrying Don.

THERAPIST: Still linked to having babies ...

CAROL: Yep, and I had plenty of that caring for my younger sibs long before I wanted to.

THERAPIST: Part of you struggles with those feelings. The rational or conscious self doesn't always go hand in hand with the old thoughts or unconscious self.

CAROL: No. It's getting better. I can sometimes recognize the struggle and talk myself through it. But not always.

THERAPIST: Are there ways you could help Don understand what you're experiencing in those moments?

DON: Sometimes I can see it, Carol. I understand it better now, and when I see you sometimes struggling when I approach you sexually, sometimes I can back off better without feeling hurt or getting angry, and wait for you eventually to get to a better place. But other times I just sense your irritation with me for wanting to have sex with you and then I retreat or lash back.

CAROL: What do you want from me, then?

DON: Well, it's like we've talked about in here before. If you're struggling, try to let me know. Just say something like "It's hard right now," rather than striking out or using your anger to push me away. I think I could use that phrase as a cue or something—you know—a signal that lets me ease up and give you some space without lashing back.

CAROL: I can try that. Sometimes I *am* irritated with you, Don, but most of the time I'm not—certainly not as often as before—but I can see I've been using the old ways of reacting to your overtures even though our relationship has changed. I'll try to recognize what's going on with me and do a better job of expressing that.

Outcome

The couple met with their therapist in conjoint sessions approximately 18 times over a 6-month period. Their levels of sexual desire never converged at the same level, but the degree of discrepancy decreased and the partners' ability to manage it improved considerably. Moreover, improvements in the couple's sexual relationship both contributed to and were strengthened by gains in other areas of their marriage—particularly in terms of communication and emotional connectedness. Two years after their treatment, the therapist ran into Don and Carol at the grocery store. By then they had a new baby in tow as well as their young toddler. They disclosed that, following her second pregnancy, Carol's depression and disruption of sexual desire had returned for several months. However, the couple had been able to review steps they had taken previously to address challenges in their marriage, and on their own had been able to restore the quality of relationship they had enjoyed earlier.

Discussion

In many respects, the diverse contributing factors to Carol's low sexual desire reported at the outset of therapy are common among couples presenting with this complaint. Similarly, the outcomes Don and Carol achieved were somewhat typical. Differences in partners' levels of sexual desire diminished but did not disappear. The couple engaged in sexual relations about three to four times per month, and both partners described the majority of these exchanges as satisfying. Although Don still would have liked to have sex more often and Carol would have been content to have it less frequently, each acknowledged and made reasonable efforts to accommodate the other's preferences. The partners' understanding of themselves and each other deepened, although each at times reenacted old patterns of responding to internal conflicts and the other's provocations. Communication patterns and overall relationship quality improved, although the marriage remained imperfect and the couple's sexual relationship would always require effort to maintain a steady flow of satisfactory exchanges. It was important to normalize this pattern for the couple and to support their efforts to find sustainable if nonpreferred compromises for the sake of their marriage.

The most important aspect of this case involves the sequencing of therapeutic interactions. It was clear from the initial assessment that Don's propensity for feeling inadequate and his impulse to retreat, and Carol's deeply conflicted feelings around her sexuality, were rooted in early developmental experiences that would eventually require explication and at least partial resolution. However, adopting a developmental approach using insight-oriented or interpretive techniques before establishing prerequisite levels of individual and relationship strength is more likely to produce iatrogenic problems than positive effects. Couples presenting with complaints of low sexual desire remain inappropriate candidates for interpretive strategies so long as they exhibit persistent hostility, mistrust, inflexibility, or resistance to change. Until an atmosphere of safety can be established that extends beyond therapy sessions to the couple's interactions outside of therapy, each individual may be reluctant to disclose the intimate and emotionally difficult material from previous relationships essential to the process of affective reconstruction of relationship themes. Both partners should exhibit some capacity for introspection, be open to examining feelings, and be able to resurrect affective experiences from previous relationships on a conscious level. Each needs to have established a basic level of trust with the therapist, experiencing the exploration of cyclical maladaptive patterns as promoting the individual's own relationship fulfillment. Moreover, both individuals need to exhibit levels of personal maturity and relationship commitment that enable them to respond to their partner's intimate disclosures with empathy and support.

COMMENTARY

For many couples, low sexual desire exists within a broader context of significant individual dysfunction in one or both partners and relationship dysfunction extending well beyond the sexual relationship. The diverse structures characterizing both the phenomenology of low sexual desire and contributing etiologies require the therapist to be theoretically and technically competent across an equally diverse range of therapeutic modalities. Effective treatment requires tailoring the selection and sequencing of interventions to the unique strengths and challenges of the individual partners, their relationship, and the broader socioecological system in which their sexual relationship is embedded. The pluralistic approach proposed here advocates examining developmental origins of partners' respective contributions to relationship struggles only after stabilizing initial individual or relational crises, directing healthier patterns of individual and couple behaviors, and promoting relationship skills involving both communication and support behaviors, which provide a foundation for more interpretive techniques. Implementing an affective reconstructive approach within the context of conjoint therapy enables partners to become more aware of and empathically responsive to each other's emotional sensitivities and struggles—including those underlying discrepant levels of sexual desire.

REFERENCES

American Psychiatric Association. (2000). *Diagnostic and statistical manual of mental disorders* (4th ed., text rev.). Washington, DC: Author.

Berg, P., & Snyder, D. K. (1981). Differential diagnosis of marital and sexual distress: A multidimensional approach. *Journal of Sex and Marital Therapy, 7,* 290–295.

Kiecolt-Glaser, J. K., & Newton, T. L. (2001). Marriage and health: His and hers. *Psychological Bulletin, 127,* 472–503.

Rodrigue, J. R., & Park, T. L. (1996). General and illness-specific adjustment to cancer: Relationship to marital status and marital quality. *Journal of Psychosomatic Research, 40,* 29–36.

Snyder, D. K. (1997). *Marital Satisfaction Inventory—Revised (MSI-R).* Los Angeles: Western Psychological Services.

Snyder, D. K. (1999). Affective reconstruction in the context of a pluralistic approach to couple therapy. *Clinical Psychology: Science and Practice, 6,* 348–365.

Snyder, D. K., Cepeda-Benito, A., Abbott, B. V., Gleaves, D. H., Negy, C., Hahlweg, K., et al. (2004). Cross-cultural applications of the Marital Satisfaction Inventory—Revised (MSI-R). In M. E. Maruish (Ed.), *Use of psychological testing for treatment planning and outcomes assessment* (3rd ed., pp. 603–623). Mahwah, NJ: Erlbaum.

Snyder, D. K., & Mitchell, A. E. (2008). Affective–reconstructive couple therapy: A pluralistic, developmental approach. In A. S. Gurman (Ed.), *Clinical handbook of couple therapy* (4th ed., pp. 353–382). New York: Guilford Press.

Snyder, D. K., & Whisman, M. A. (2003). *Treating difficult couples: Helping clients with coexisting mental and relationship disorders.* New York: Guilford Press.

Snyder, D. K., & Whisman, M. A. (2004, November). Comorbid relationship and individual distress: Challenges for intervention and research. In E. Lawrence (Chair), *Adapting the theme of comorbidity to the study of intimate relationships.* Symposium presented at the meeting of the Association for Behavioral and Cognitive Therapies, New Orleans, LA.

Whisman, M. A. (2006). Role of couples' relationships in understanding and treating mental disorders. In S. R. H. Beach, M. Z. Wamboldt, N. J. Kaslow, R. E. Heyman, M. B. First, L. G. Underwood, et al. (Eds.), *Relational processes and DSM-V: Neuroscience, assessment, prevention, and treatment* (pp. 225–238). Washington, DC: American Psychiatric Association.

Chapter 12

The Role of Androgens in the Treatment of Hypoactive Sexual Desire Disorder in Women

Joanna B. Korda
Sue W. Goldstein
Irwin Goldstein

Most of the chapters in this book have focused on treating sexual desire complaints in a psychological or relationship context. In this informative chapter, Joann B. Korda, Sue W. Goldstein, and Irwin Goldstein describe the role of androgens specifically testosterone, in the treatment of primary hypoactive sexual desire disorder (HSDD) in a young woman about to be married.

A thorough physical exam and vascular and hormonal evaluation of the client reveals significant evidence of hormonal insufficiency, evidenced by labial resorption and mild genital sensory neuropathy, as well as long-standing sexual complaints. The authors speculate that the low androgen levels have led to cerebral changes in the patient's neurotransmitters, resulting in diminished sexual desire as well as changes in the structure of the genital organs—all of which have interfered with the ability to respond physically to sexual stimulation.

The case described is a challenging one in that it involves the primary lack of sexual desire as well as concomitant difficulties with arousal, orgasm, and sexual pain. The authors provide a persuasive discussion of the importance of adequate hormonal function for sexual satisfaction and function. With the use of systemic testosterone, local estradiol, and a systemic dopamine agonist, as well as several sessions of more traditional sex therapy, the client reported significant improvement in all areas of her sexual life. While she remains anorgasmic at the conclusion of treatment, she is pleased with the treatment outcome and expresses a desire to remain on hormonal therapy.

This case illustrates the importance of undertaking a thorough medical and hormonal as well as psychological and interpersonal evaluation in individuals experiencing lifelong as well as acquired sexual complaints.

Joanna B. Korda, MD, is a research scholar at San Diego State University and a clinical research fellow at San Diego Sexual Medicine.

Sue W. Goldstein, BA, is the program and clinical research coordinator at San Diego Sexual Medicine.

Irwin Goldstein, MD, is the Director of Sexual Medicine at Alvarado Hospital in San Diego. He is admired and respected for his tireless and effective efforts to position sexual medicine as a major health discipline as well as his success in launching and serving as editor-in-chief of *The Journal of Sexual Medicine.*

The authors work in a multidisciplinary facility consisting of a physician, a sex therapist, and support personnel. As a medical office, we may have a patient population that differs from that of a psychologist's office. The most common complaint of women seeking consultation at our clinic is secondary hypoactive sexual desire disorder (HSDD). Often, this is associated with the aftermath of childbirth, menopause, and the use of oral contraceptives or antidepressants. The preportion of men complaining of HSDD is significantly lower, approximately 10%. Women often come to our clinic because of their feelings of guilt about denying a partner sex or fears of losing a partner because of the lack of sexual intimacy. They also present because they are distressed over their inability to feel the desire they once had.

WHAT IS SEXUAL DESIRE?

Sexual desire, the mental state of fantasy about and interest in sexual activity, is under the control of both the autonomic and somatic nervous systems. Neurotransmitters such as dopamine, noradrenaline, melanocortin, and oxytocin are important for sexual response and interest. They are excitatory and act on the limbic system and hypothalamic regions. Sexual inhibition is mediated by other neurotransmitters, namely, serotonin, cerebral opioids, and endocannabinoids (Pfais. 2008; Giuliano, Rampin, & Allard, 2002; Clayton, 2007). The sexual excitatory pathway is stimulated hormonally by steroid hormones—estrogens, androgens, and progestins. Natural or medically or surgically induced hormone deficiency is often accompanied by a loss of interest in sex and reduced responsiveness to sexual stimuli.

This chapter provides a brief overview of the biological basis of HSDD secondary to androgen deficiency and illustrates how the addition of testosterone was helpful in the treatment of a young woman presenting with both lack of desire and long-standing difficulties experiencing subjective sexual arousal.

CASE EXAMPLE: REMI

Remi is a 25-year-old woman who was engaged to be married in 3 months. She complained of a lifelong history of absent sexual desire and arousal. Her concerns about embarking on a marriage in this state as well as the realization that she was not alone with this problem led her to seek help. When first seen, she reported feeling sexually indifferent, apathetic, pessimistic, and impatient with and disappointed in her overall sexual life.

Past History

Remi grew up in a loving and caring atmosphere. Her parents, both atheists, were teachers and provided a safe and loving family environment, as Remi stated when we first met her. Her earliest sexual memory was from the age of 13 when her first boyfriend, with whom she thought she was in love, wanted to kiss her. She experienced sexual thoughts and fantasies, but did not feel the desire or need to masturbate, and therefore has never done so. At the age of 14 she began to kiss boys and found she liked it, but she experienced little pleasure from kissing. During the following years she engaged in sexual intimacy with boyfriends only because of "peer pressure."

She had oral sex at age 16 and intercourse at age 17 with a 26-year-old married high school teacher. She said it was primarily a sense of curiosity that drew her to have with sex with him, although it was not totally consensual. She hoped to experience sexual excitement and pleasure with a more sexually experienced partner, although this did not happen for Remi. Over a period of 3 months, she had intercourse several times before she ended the sexual relationship with the teacher. The following two relationships prior to her engagement failed because of her lack of sexual desire.

Remi has been with her current partner for 3 years and describes him as loving, caring, and understanding. Her partner initiates sexual activity about once a week. He is supportive and does not pressure her. She wishes to feel sexual desire and also to feel more during sexual activity. A brief course of sex therapy in the past failed to improve her desire for sex. She does not report a history of depression, anxiety, obsessive–compulsive disorder, or other mood disorders.

Medical History

Remi started menstruating at the age of 13. She used oral contraception for 4 years, followed by a contraceptive patch at the age of 18, and noted decreasing lubrication during sexual activity with both. Currently, she does not use hormonal contraception. Notable in her history was the fact that Remi had fallen off horses several times in the past, injuring her perineal area when she was kicked. She had sought medical help in the past to overcome her sexual complaints. Previous hormonal blood testing and an evaluation for pudendal nerve entrapment showed no abnormal findings. She was seen by a sex therapist to rule out any negative impact from her sexual relationship with her high school teacher. She was made aware of the imbalance in maturity and power in this relationship because of the age and status differences between the two of them. After a few sessions with the sex therapist, she did not experience any improvement in her sexual function, so she stopped going.

Remi's diagnosis is primary female HSDD, primary orgasmic disorder, and secondary sexual pain disorder.

Diagnosis

To assess possible biological causes of sexual dysfunction, all female patients in our sexual medicine facility undergo the same diagnostic paradigm consisting of physical examination including vulvoscopy, quantitative sensory testing using biothesiometry and hot and cold temperature testing, duplex Doppler ultrasound, and blood tests.

Physical Examination and Vulvoscopy

Vulvoscopy is a procedure for examining a woman's vestibular region under a microscope. Remi's examination revealed pathology consistent with bilateral labial resorption of her labia minora (they were actually disappearing) with absence of the lower third of the labia in the area of the posterior fourchette. Furthermore the bilateral superior vestibular glands, which are located at the vaginal opening, showed erythema, or redness and tenderness, and she experienced 3 out of 10 and 6 out of 10 pain with Q-Tip testing. These local, genital physical findings are typically seen in women affected by a hormonal deficiency. Local estrogen deficiency leads to resorption of the labia minora (Leung, Robson, Kao, Liu, & Fong, 2005). Testosterone deficiency is one of the major causes of pain and erythema of the vestibular glands, as was evident with Remi (Bouchard, Brisson, Fortier, Morin, & Blanchette, 2002).

Blood Tests

Hormone blood values are measured in every patient presenting to our facility to rule out hormonal dysfunction known to be a common cause of sexual health complaints. To assess the function of the pituitary gland, we determine the levels of thyroid-stimulating hormone (TSH), luteinizing (LH) and follicle-stimulating (FSH) hormones and prolactin. To evaluate the function of the ovaries and adrenal glands, we determine the levels of estradiol, progesterone, and two of the major androgens, dihydrotestosterone (DHT) and total testosterone. To complete our assessment of the important blood values we determine the level of sex-hormone-binding globulin (SHBG). To rule out bias within the testosterone determination, we calculate the value of the free, bioavailable, and therefore active testosterone ourselves, using the free testosterone calculator (*www.issam.ch/freetests.htm*) rather than relying on the blood test.

We encourage every professional interested in sexual health to measure hormone blood levels. The results of these multiple tests need to be examined very carefully. Usually a pattern will emerge that helps in recommending a course of action. It is generally agreed that a hormone blood level in the lowest fourth or quartile of the normal range is considered suspicious. The rationale behind this principle is that laboratories developed current values for the "normal range" by measuring hormone blood values of healthy women without knowledge of the women's sexual function. Thus the so-called "normal range" may not reflect sexual health and may include women who were not sexually healthy. Women's blood test values have now been examined in several studies that excluded women with health concerns, including sexual health concerns (Guay et al., 2004).

Remi's blood test results revealed a low value of testosterone, consistent with testosterone deficiency (see Table 12.1).

Neurological Testing

Biothesiometry, which measures vibration perception thresholds, showed a vibration perception threshold of 3 volts in the pulp of Remi's right index finger (nongenital site used as baseline) and a mildly increased vibration perception threshold of 6 volts in her clitoris, and left and right labia minora. Temperature testing is another valuable methodology to assess neurological function of the external genitalia. Since heat and cold are felt by different receptors, both are measured. Temperature testing showed an elevated heat perception threshold in Remi's genital area with 30°C in her index finger, 35°C in her clitoris, and 37°C in her right and left labia minora, and an elevated cold perception threshold in her genital area with 20°C in her index finger, 18°C in her clitoris, and 12°C in her right and left labia minora. This quantitative sensory testing, using biothesiometry and hot and cold temperature testing, revealed a mild to moderate sensory neuropathy

TABLE 12.1. Remi´s Blood Test Results at Her First Visit, before Treatment

	Value	Reference range (RR)	RR follicular phase	RR midcycle phase	RR luteal phase
TSH	0.62 mIU/ml	0.47–4.68			
LH	5.3 mIU/ml		1.9–12.5	8.7–76.3	0.5–16.9
FSH	4.2 mIU/ml		2.5–10.2	3.1–17.7	1.5–9.1
Prolactin	6.4 ng/ml	3–30			
Estradiol (E2)	39 pg/ml		27–161	187–382	33–201
Progesterone	0.39 ng/ml		0.12–1.7		
0.39–5.88	1.02–22.4				
DHEA-S	42 mcg/dl	45–320			
Total testosterone	21 ng/dl	20–76			
SHBG	69 nmol/l	6–112			

Note. Reference range is that of healthy premenopausal women.

of the vestibule consistent with the weakened genital sensations that Remi had described previously.

Duplex Doppler Ultrasonography

The purpose of performing duplex Doppler ultrasonography is to visualize vascular structures in a noninvasive manner to see whether blood flow is normal or not. Remi had adequate increases in peak systolic velocity of the right and left cavernosal arteries. There was no evidence of clitoral fibrosis or inhomogeneity of the erectile tissue, and her arousal response was adequate. We were therefore able to rule out any pathological changes in the structure of her external sexual organs or in the blood supply to her external genitals. There was no sign of a vascular origin of her sexual complaints.

Summary of Physical Findings

In summary, Remi was diagnosed with HSDD, arousal and orgasmic disorder, and dyspareunia. On physical examination there was mild genital sensory neuropathy, bilateral labial resorption, and adenitis of the anterior vestibular glands at 1 and 11 o'clock. These abnormal physical findings are commonly associated with a hormonal insufficiency, in particular, decreased testosterone levels. This finding of androgen deficiency was supported by her blood test results, which revealed insufficient testosterone levels. Our patient Remi was found to have biologically induced sexual dysfunction secondary to low testosterone. The low testosterone led to changes in the cerebral neurotransmitters that decreased her sexual desire and to changes in the morphology or structure of her genital organs, leading to a dysfunctional physical response to sexual stimulation (Pfaus, 2008; Giuliano, Rampin, & Allard, 2002; Clayton, 2007).

Androgens

Androgens are often considered the "hormones of desire." They consist of seven different sex steroids that are naturally synthesized from cholesterol by the ovaries and the adrenal gland, and from other androgens in peripheral organs such as skeletal muscle and skin. While all seven androgens are important for tissue structure and function, four of the seven are often clinically measured: dehydroepiandrosterone (DHEA), androstenedione, testosterone, and DHT.

DHEA, the first or precursor androgen, is converted by an enzyme into androstenedione, which is then converted by a different enzyme into testosterone, which in turn is converted by yet another enzyme to DHT. Studies have shown that 90% of the DHEA is synthesized in the adrenal gland, with the remaining 10% synthesized in the ovaries (Labrie, Luu-The, Labrie, & Simard, 2001; Bachmann et al., 2002).

Androgens have an effect on many physiological functions in women including (1) stimulation of sexual desire, interest, thoughts, and fantasies; (2) regulation of genital (vaginal and clitoral) blood flow, amount and quality of vaginal lubrication, and structural and functional integrity of the clitoris, prepuce, vagina, and minor vestibular glands; (3) stimulation of bone growth; (4) increase in muscle mass; (5) maintenance of energy and well-being; (6) maintenance of lean body composition; (7) control of oil gland activity in skin; and (8) regulation of body hair growth (Traish, Kim, Min, Munarriz, & Goldstein, 2002; Traish, Kim, Stankovic, Goldstein, & Kim, 2007).

The level of circulating androgens in women declines with age, beginning at about age 30 and continuing with each passing decade. For example, at age 40, a woman's testosterone values are half what they were at age 20, and at age 60, the testosterone values are one-third of the values at age 20. In addition to aging, there are other conditions or situations associated with lower testosterone blood levels. The most common is an elevation in SHBG. The purpose of SHBG is to bind the sex steroids (androgens, estrogens, and progestins) in the circulation. With sex steroids in general and testosterone specifically, it is the "free" form, not the "bound" form, that is physiologically active. SHBG values are increased by use of any synthetic estrogen (e.g., oral, patch, or ring contraceptives, or estrogens for treatment of menopausal symptoms), by tamoxifen (for breast cancer), and by pregnancy, liver diseases such as cirrhosis, and some antiseizure medications, all of which result in less "free" testosterone. SHBG is lowered by androgen administration, a bonus of testosterone use. Low androgen levels are associated with any condition, treatment, or type of birth control that affects the ovary, such as natural, surgical, or premature menopause; injury to the ovary by chemotherapy or radiation treatments for cancer; oral, patch, or ring contraceptives; infertility, or hormone treatments for endometriosis, or uterine fibroids (Panzer et al., 2006).

The following symptoms may indicate androgen deficiency: (1) a diminished sense of well-being, (2) feeling helpless or unhappy, (3) having persistent or unexplained fatigue, (4) experiencing sexual function changes such as decreased sexual interest, receptivity, or pleasure, and/or decreased lubrication, (5) bone loss, decreased muscle strength, or changes of memory (Brown, 2008; Kingsberg, 2007; Morsink et al., 2007; Schwenkhagen, 2007). Before considering a diagnosis such as depression or another psychological condition, we strongly recommend assessing for hormonal insufficiency or other biological causes of sexual health complaints.

Therapy

Remi was advised to begin sex therapy to deal with her fear of losing her partner due to her lack of sexual desire, and to initiate strategies such as directed masturbation and vibrator therapy. Directed masturbation is very helpful in showing a woman how to experience and appreciate physical reactions to sexual stimulation outside the context of sexual activity with another person. In women diagnosed with sensory neuropathy, it is very valuable to encourage masturbation with a vibrator that is strong enough to stimulate a sufficient genital arousal response. That kind of therapy is not only educational but can improve genital morphology secondary to the increase in blood supply to the clitoris and vagina.

In addition to sex therapy Remi was advised to consider hormonal treatment. This included (1) systemic testosterone, (2) local estradiol to the labia minora and the vestibule, and (3) a systemic dopamine agonist. Currently there are no hormone therapies approved by the Food and Drug Administration (FDA) for women with sexual health problems except for vaginal atrophy. This means that the safety and/or efficacy of androgen use in women with sexual health problems has not yet been satisfactorily established. This type of androgen use is currently considered "off-label" treatment. It is important for health care providers to inform their patients of this and provide them with appropriate evidence-based information on the risks and benefits of each proposed medication. Each patient should be able to make an educated decision as to the potential use of each off-label medication. Remi asked about the data relating to adverse effects of testosterone therapy. For testosterone, recognized concerns involve (1) hirsutism, acne, and virilization; (2) cardiovascular issues and abnormal effects on lipids, erythrocytes, blood viscosity, and blood coagulation; (3) breast cancer; (4) stimulation of the uterine lining; and (5) liver function changes, sleep apnea, and aggression (Boulour & Braunstein, 2005; Shufelt & Braunstein, 2009).

A total of 3–8% of women using testosterone for management of sexual health problems noted side effects. They were usually mild and dependent upon dose and duration of treatment. Virilization could occur with the high testosterone doses required for management of female-to-male transsexuals, but at the low doses used to treat women with sexual dysfunction, it is exceedingly rare. Even at the high doses used in the management of female-to-male transsexuals, testosterone use has not been linked to an increase in vascular deaths or deterioration in vascular health including heart attack, chest pain, or increased blood pressure. Women who used testosterone showed no difference from placebo in data regarding abnormal changes in lipids, erythrocytes, blood viscosity, or blood coagulation (Shufelt & Braunstein, 2009).

There are fears concerning breast cancer because androgen receptors are present in the breast cells. Breast stromal (not ductal) tissue has the ability to undergo aromatization of testosterone to estradiol, and some studies suggest a relationship between high testosterone and breast cancer, but the significance of the data is questioned. Of note, however, there is no increased risk of breast cancer in women who have elevated testosterone from polycystic ovary disease. In multiple studies, testosterone use shows no increase in breast cancer risk, and in many studies, one can infer that testosterone may actually be protective. Breast cancer potential was measured in monkeys using an index of breast tissue proliferation (Shufelt & Braunstein, 2009; Bitzer, Kenemans, Mueck, & FSD Education Group, 2008). In those treated with estradiol alone, the breast tissue proliferation was four times that in the control animals. In those animals co-treated with estradiol and testosterone, the risk was one-half that group treated with the estradiol alone (Dauvois, Geng, Lévesque, Mérand, & Labrie, 1991). In a breast cancer comparison study, the cases of breast cancer per 100,000 women-years in women using estrogen and testosterone or estrogen, progesterone, and testosterone were lower than in women using estrogen and progesterone (Dimitrakakis, Jones, Liu, & Bondy, 2004). Of note, whereas many studies show no increase in breast cancer in women using bioidentical testosterone, a recent study of nurses showed that those who used the nonbioidentical form of testosterone called methyl testosterone in conjunction with a fixed dose of estradiol did indeed have a higher risk of breast cancer compared to those who used the bioidentical form of testosterone (Tamimi, Hankinson, Chen, Rosner, & Colditz, 2006).

We use bioidentical products that are FDA approved (for other indications) whenever possible. After we discussed the pros and cons of each medication, Remi was prescribed testosterone, local estradiol, and a dopamine agonist. The testosterone gel is FDA approved for men. She was advised to apply it daily to her calves at one-tenth the amount prescribed for a man. Individual doses of testosterone are best established by repeated follow-up blood tests of total testosterone and SHBG, usually at 3-month intervals.

A wide selection of topical estradiol products is available. It is very important to acknowledge the outstanding resorptive capacity of the vaginal tissue, leading to an increase in systemic hormonal values depending on the administered dose, which requires repeated follow-up. Remi decided to use estradiol cream, which she was advised to apply daily on her vestibule and labia minora, as well as her clitoral region. In addition, Remi started taking bupropion, one of several available dopamine agonists. She was placed on 75-mg bupropion tablets daily, the most common choice in our clinic.

Outcome of Treatment

After 3 months of treatment including sex therapy, daily testosterone gel, daily estrogen cream, and daily bupropion administration, Remi noted a marked improvement in her sexual function. She reported initiating sexual activity and feeling sexual desire, and lubrication and genital engorgement occurred more rapidly. She also noted improved genital sensation and reported regular involuntary muscle contractions during sexual activity. Unfortunately she remained unable to experience orgasm during sexual stimulation, but she had only been on treatment for 3 months. She did not experience any negative side effects associated with the androgen treatment,

At 6-months follow-up Remi showed a significant improvement on a validated questionnaire, the Female Sexual Function Inventory (FSFI), from baseline at her first visit. Both her FSFI total score and the individual domain scores improved with the exception of orgasm, indicating that she had experienced a significant improvement of her sexuality. The physical examination, including vulvoscopy and quantitative sensory testing, also revealed significant improvement. During the vulvoscopic examination the labial resorption in the fourchette area was remarkably reduced, and both labia minora showed less resorption. The vestibular glands did not show any erythema or tenderness. Her vibration thresholds improved to 4 volts for index finger and clitoris and 5 volts for her labia minora. The heat and cold perception threshold values also improved. This showed measurable improvement in the sensory function of her nerve structures as well as a change in the morphology of the labia minora and the vestibule. In support of these physical findings, which indicate an increase in systemic androgen and local estrogen levels, the calculated free testosterone was 0.84 ng/dl (reference range: 0.6–0.8). We are currently exploring other avenues, including oral administration of oxytocin, to improve her orgasmic function.

COMMENTARY

While there are numerous psychological and biological pathophysiologies for HSDD, in this chapter we have focused on HSDD secondary to androgen deficiency syndrome, as illustrated through Remi's case report.

The central and peripheral sexual function response, which includes the mental state of sexual desire and arousal as well as the physical response of the genitals, needs an intact hormonal system. Steroid hormones are critical for (1) the priming of the brain to be selectively responsive to sexual stimuli and (2) maintaining the health and function of the genital tissue involved in the sexual response.

To prime the brain for selective responses to sexual stimulation, excitatory neurotransmitters and their receptors are synthesized in the central nervous system. The synthesis of excitatory neurotransmitters (dopamine, noradrenaline, melanocortin, and oxytocin) is mediated in part by steroid hormones. There are numerous examples in the literature of the hormonal relationship to sexual desire (Chudakov, Ben Zion, & Belmaker, 2007; Clayton, 2007; Giuliano, Rampin, & Allard, 2002; Kingsberg, 2007; Pfaus, 2008). Androgen deprivation states, as seen in women after ovariectomy and adrenalectomy, are commonly accompanied by a loss of libido and decreased sexual activity. There are a large number of double-blind, placebo-controlled trials in postmenopausal women diagnosed with HSDD showing the restoration of sexual function and desire after testosterone therapy (Kingsberg, 2007).

Steroidogenic enzymes in the peripheral genital tissue synthesize androgens and estrogens locally intracellular from the adrenal precursors DHEA and androstenedione. Estrogens modulate peripheral genital hemodynamics and are critical for the structural and functional integrity of the vaginal tissue (Giraldi et al., 2004). Estrogen deprivation results in atrophic changes in the vaginal mucosa, thinning of the epithelium, loss of vaginal rugae, reduction of vaginal lubrication, and fusion of the labia. The sensory function of the vulvar epithelium is known to improve in response to hormone therapy. Local genital androgen and estrogen deficiency does not just lead to a disruption in vaginal epithelial morphology and function, but may secondarily affect intraepithelial nerve fibers, resulting in a decrease of genital sensory function (Alatas, Yagei, Oztekin, & Sabir, 2008; Traish, Kim, Min, Munarriz, & Goldstein, 2002; Traish, Kim, Stankovic, Goldstein, & Kim, 2007).

There are several research studies reporting a positive correlation between low libido and an insufficient genital response to sexual stimulation (Basson, 2001; Basson, Brotto, Laan, Redmond, & Utian, 2005; Carvalho & Nobre, 2010). Considering the testosterone dependency of genital tissue and regulation of genital smooth muscle tone, we believe in a dual, interdependent mechanism of action. Testosterone increases subjective (central) and peripheral (genital) arousal. Physical pleasure facilitates sexual desire. A poor genital response leads to frustration and disappointment and inhibits sexual desire.

Both animal and human studies have shown alterations in genital hemodynamics after testosterone treatment. Tuiten et al. (2002) demonstrated statistically significant enhancement of vaginal blood flow response to visual erotic stimuli after sublingual testosterone administration in healthy women. The increase in vaginal blood flow was accompanied by an increase in subjective genital arousal and sexual lust (Tuiten, van Honk, Verbaten, Laan, Everaerd, & Stam, 2002).

The positive effect of testosterone therapy in premenopausal women affected by HSDD has been shown in a number of studies. These results are in accord with our experience with Remi as well as our daily observations in our sexual medicine clinic concerning beneficial therapeutic outcomes with testosterone treatment in pre- and postmenopausal women diagnosed with HSDD with low androgen levels.

The testosterone deficiency in our patient led to a decrease in her desire for sexual activity in at least two ways. One part was the change of cerebral mediators, in fact excitatory neurotransmitters, which are important in priming the brain to develop sexual desire and be open and responsive to sexual stimuli. The other important part was the change in her genitals, leading to a dysfunction of the genital tissue itself with changes of the labia minora and vestibule and also of the sensory function of her genital area, so she was not able to react in a healthy and pleasurable way to sexual stimulation. We also believe that the weak physical reaction resulted in a negative change in psychological status and reaction, comparable to a negative feedback mechanism from her body to the brain.

How did our patient, Remi, develop androgen insufficiency syndrome along with local genital estrogen insufficiency, leading to her sexual complaints? We believe the key to this answer was her choice of hormonal contraception versus mechanical contraception, since she did not have a surgically or naturally induced hormonal dysfunction. Ethinyl estradiol, a synthetic estrogen often combined with a synthetic progesterone, is the common ingredient found in all hormonal contraceptives. Ethinyl estradiol is 600 times more potent for the estradiol receptor than the bioidentical 17 beta-estradiol. Use of ethinyl estradiol leads to diminished FSH and LH, the pituitary hormones that act on the ovaries, and reduced ovarian metabolic activity with decreased circulating levels of androgens and estrogens and marked increase in hepatic synthesis of SHBG, the major binding protein for sex steroid hormones in the circulation. Oral contraceptive–induced hormonal modifications result in alteration of androgen hormone levels, particularly in low levels of free and bioavailable testosterone. The most common reported side effects include diminished sexual interest, decreased frequency of sexual intercourse, diminished vaginal lubrication, decreased sexual arousal, and increased pain during intercourse (Panzer et al., 2006; Warnock et al., 2006).

Use of synthetic estrogens for contraception results in two problems. First, the ovaries, the main producers of estrogens, progesterone, and androgens in premenopausal women, shut down as a negative feedback mechanism. For Remi, the problem was that with her oral contraception she had a supply of estrogen and progesterone but not of androgen, since most oral contraceptives have very low or no androgenic activity. Women using oral contraception provoke androgen insufficiency by shutting down their own production of steroid hormones in the ovaries. The second important contributor to low androgen levels was the fact that the estrogen Remi was taking was a synthetic estrogen (ethinyl estrogen). Her liver was trying to rid her body of the foreign substance and therefore increased the synthesis of SHBG, binding the remaining steroid hormones in her blood, which resulted in another decrease of free, active androgens.

The androgen insufficiency led to a disruption in the functional integrity of the vestibule, vagina, and clitoris, resulting in inflammation of the vestibular glands and therefore pain during intercourse. This was the third contributing factor to Remi's HSDD and anorgasmia (Bouchard et al., 2002; Greenstein et al., 2007).

In summary, androgen deprivation may alter neurotransmitters and their receptors as well as genital tissue integrity and function. Taking into account that desire and arousal are dependent on the balance and integration of multiple physiological systems controlled by neurotransmitters, vasoactive agents, and endocrine factors and require a functional and healthy tissue structure of the genital sexual organs, it is easy to understand how the pathophysiology of androgen deficiency can lead to HSDD in women and men.

Our patient, Remi, experienced improved sexual function while on testosterone treatment and wishes to remain on the treatment.

CONCLUSION

What is the bottom line? DHEA and testosterone are critical sex steroids for sexual function and structure in women and men. New clinical studies of safety and efficacy data for the judicious use of bioidentical testosterone continue to be gathered and are available for all patients (and partners) and health care providers to analyze. Each individual must weigh the risks and benefits of using these sex steroids to treat androgen insufficiency. For those who decide the benefits outweigh the risks, the most prudent plan is to use bioidentical testosterone in doses that maintain hormone values in an appropriate physiological range, undergo frequent and regular blood testing, and undergo routine breast exams, mammograms, and gynecological exams.

While our understanding of the *biological* mechanisms of sexual desire, arousal, and orgasm is still unfolding, it is hoped that researchers and clinicians alike understand that sexual desire—both its stimulation and inhibition—is indeed *biologically* "in the head."

REFERENCES

Alatas, E., Yagci B., Oztekin, O., & Sabir, N. (2008). Effect of hormone replacement therapy on clitoral artery blood flow in healthy postmenopausal women. *Journal of Sexual Medicine, 5*, 2367–2373.

Bachmann. G., Bancroft, J., Braunstein, G., Burger, H., Davis, S., Dennerstein, L., et al. (2002). Female androgen insufficiency: The Princeton consensus statement on definition, classification, and assessment. *Fertility and Sterility, 77*, 660–665.

Basson, R. (2001). Human sex-response cycles. *Journal of Sex and Marital Therapy, 27*, 33–43.

Basson, R., Brotto, L. A., Laan, E., Redmond, G., & Utian, W. H. (2005). Assessment and management of women's sexual dysfunctions: Problematic desire and arousal. *Journal of Sexual Medicine, 2*, 291–300.

Bitzer, J., Kenemans, P., Mueck, A. O., & FSD Education Group. (2008). Breast cancer risk in postmenopausal women using testosterone in combination with hormone replacement therapy. *Maturitas, 59*, 209–218.

Bolour, S., & Braunstein, G. (2005). Testosterone therapy in women: A review. *International Journal of Impotence Research, 17*, 399–408.

Bouchard, C., Brisson, J., Fortier, M., Morin, C., & Blanchette C. (2002). Use of oral contraceptive pills and vulvar vestibulitis: A case-control study. *American Journal of Epidemiology, 156*, 254–261.

Brown, M. (2008). Skeletal muscle and bone: Effect of sex steroids and aging. *Advances in Physiology Education, 32*, 120–126.

Carvalho, J., & Nobre, P. (2010). Predictors of women's sexual desire: The role of psychopathology, cognitive-emotional determinants, relationship dimensions, and medical factors. *Journal of Sexual Medicine, 7*, 928–937.

Chudakov, B., Ben Zion, I. Z., & Belmaker, R. H. (2007). Transdermal testosterone gel prn application for hypoactive sexual desire disorder in premenopausal women: A controlled pilot study of the effects on the Arizona Sexual Experiences Scale for females and sexual function questionnaire. *Journal of Sexual Medicine, 4*, 204–208.

Clayton, A. H. (2007). Epidemiology and neurobiology of female sexual dysfunction. *Journal of Sexual Medicine, 4*, S260–S268.

Dauvois, S., Geng, C. S., Lévesque, C., Mérand, Y., & Labrie, F. (1991). Additive inhibitory effects of an androgen and the antiestrogen EM-170 on estradiol-stimulated growth of human ZR-75-1 breast tumors in athymic mice. *Cancer Research, 51*, 3131–3135.

Dimitrakakis, C., Jones, R. A., Liu, A., & Bondy, C. A. (2004). Breast cancer incidence in postmenopausal women using testosterone in addition to usual hormone therapy. *Menopause, 11*, 531–535.

Giraldi, A., Marson, L., Nappi, R., Pfaus, J., Traish, A. M., Vardi, Y., et al.(2004). Physiology of female sexual function: Animal models. *Journal of Sexual Medicine, 1*, 237–253.

Giuliano, F., Rampin, O., & Allard, J. (2002). Neurophysiology and pharmacology of female genital sexual response. *Journal of Sex and Marital Therapy, 28*, 101–121.

Greenstein, A., Ben-Aroya, Z., Fass, O., Militscher, I., Roslik, Y., Chen, J., et al. (2007). Vulvar vestibulitis syndrome and estrogen dose of oral contraceptive pills. *Journal of Sexual Medicine, 4*, 1679–1683.

Guay, A., Munarriz, R., Jacobson, J., Talakoub, L., Traish, A., Quirk, F., et al. (2004). Serum androgen levels in healthy premenopausal women with and without sexual dysfunction: Part A. Serum androgen levels in women aged 20–49 years with no complaints of sexual dysfunction. *International Journal of Impotence Research, 16*, 112–120.

Kingsberg, S. (2007). Testosterone treatment for hypoactive sexual desire disorder in postmenopausal women. *Journal of Sexual Medicine, 4*, S227–S234.

Labrie, F., Luu-The, V., Labrie, C., & Simard, J. (2001). DHEA and its transformation into androgens and estrogens in peripheral target tissues: Intracrinology. *Frontiers in Neuroendocrinology, 22*, 185–212.

Leung, A. K., Robson, W. L., Kao, C. P., Liu, E. K., & Fong, J. H. (2005). Treatment of labial fusion with topical estrogen therapy. *Clinical Pediatrics, 44*, 245–247.

Morsink, L. F., Vogelzangs, N., Nicklas, B. J., Beekman, A. T., Satterfield, S., & Rubin, S. M. (2007). Associations between sex steroid hormone levels and depressive symptoms in elderly men and women: Results from the Health ABC study. *Psychoneuroendocrinology, 32*, 874–883.

Panzer, C., Wise, S., Fantini, G., Kang, D., Munarriz, R., Guay, A., et al. (2006). Impact of oral contraceptives on sex hormone-binding globulin and androgen levels: A retrospective study in women with sexual dysfunction. *Journal of Sexual Medicine, 3*, 104–113.

Pfaus, J. (2008). The vermin that help us. *Journal of Sexual Medicine, 5*, 253–256.

Schwenkhagen, A. (2007). Hormonal changes in menopause and implications on sexual health. *Journal of Sexual Medicine, 4*, S220–S226.

Shufelt, C. L., & Braunstein, G. D. (2009). Safety of testosterone use in women. *Maturitas, 63*, 63–66.

Tamimi, R. M., Hankinson, S. E., Chen, W. Y., Rosner, B., & Colditz, G. A. (2006). Combined estrogen and testosterone use and risk of breast cancer in postmenopausal women. *Archives of Internal Medicine, 166*, 1483–1489.

Traish, A. M., Kim, N., Min, K., Munarriz, R., & Goldstein, I. (2002). Role of androgens in female genital sexual arousal: Receptor expression, structure, and function. *Fertility and Sterility, 77*, S11–S18.

Traish, A. M., Kim, S. W., Stankovic, M., Goldstein, I., & Kim, N. N. (2007). Testosterone increases blood flow and expression of androgen and estrogen receptors in the rat vagina. *Journal of Sexual Medicine, 4*, 609–619.

Tuiten, A., van Honk, J., Verbaten, R., Laan, E., Everaerd, W., & Stam, H. (2002). Can sublingual testosterone increase subjective and physiological measures of laboratory-induced sexual arousal? *Archives of General Psychiatry, 59*, 465–466.

van der Made, F., Bloemers, J., Yassem, W. E., Kleiverda, G., Everaerd, W., van Ham, D., et al. (2009). The influence of testosterone combined with a PDE5-inhibitor on cognitive, affective, and physiological sexual functioning in women suffering from sexual dysfunction. *Journal of Sexual Medicine, 6,* 777–790.

Warnock, J. K., Clayton, A., Croft, H., Segraves, R., & Biggs, F. C. (2006). Comparison of androgens in women with hypoactive sexual desire disorder: Those on combined oral contraceptives (COCs) vs. those not on COCs. *Journal of Sexual Medicine, 3,* 878–882.

Chapter 13

Sexual Psychopharmacology and Treatment of Desire Deregulation

Bonnie R. Saks

While there has always been a search for a "perfect" drug that might stimulate sexual desire or enhance sexual pleasure, the sad fact is that no such pill exists. Nevertheless, the addition of well-chosen medications can play an important role in the management of sexual problems. Certainly, many men with erectile problems have benefited greatly from the availability of the phosphodiesterase (PDE5) inhibitors, such as tadalafil, sildenafil, and vardenafil (e.g., Cialis, Viagra, and Levitra). Often these are first-line interventions for men with organic erectile dysfunction. Unfortunately, these medications do little to enhance sexual desire.

The majority of cases in this book deal with low or absent sexual interest. However, often the problem is not with too little sexual interest, but rather with too much. For such individuals, sexual psychopharmacology can be an important adjunct to treatment.

In this chapter, Bonnie R. Saks describes a unique case in which both wife and husband report sexual behaviors that detract from their marital relationship and reflect a reliance on sex to distract from, or attempt to deal with, unfinished issues stemming from childhood. Sally engages in multiple affairs to seek affirmation of her desirability, and Richard uses pornography and prostitutes to deal with underlying feelings of inadequacy and to cope with periods of stress or anxiety. Both have "addictive personalities" and a past history of substance abuse. Psychotherapy alone is ineffective in reducing their sexual impulsivity, yet finding the right medication that controls, but does not destroy, their sexual function is challenging.

Displaying an impressive knowledge of pharmacology and genuine empathy in working with both Sally and Richard, Saks determines the most efficacious medications with the fewest negative side effects. In this and similar cases the thoughtful adjunctive use of medications can provide biochemical support that facilitates a positive therapeutic outcome.

Bonnie R. Saks, MD, is a Clinical Professor of Psychiatry at the University of South Florida, Tampa, and Managing Partner of Bonnie R. Saks, MD, and Associates, LLC, a multidisciplinary group of psychopharmacologists and therapists. She is the Immediate Past President (2007–2009) of the Society for Sex Therapy and Research.

DEVELOPMENT AND FOCUS OF DESIRE

Sexual desire is a complex phenomenon influenced by early developmental (usually parental) models and attachments, social, cultural, and religious beliefs and taboos, comfort with and control of one's body, and relationships, past and present. Sexual urges are also affected by physiological and biochemical factors, both internal and externally introduced. Sexual desire is a normal and natural phenomenon, usually involving another adult person or persons. Sometimes sexual desire deviates toward a paraphilic (e.g., fetishistic, non-adult, or nonhuman) object or toward oneself (autogynophilic) or is displaced or absent altogether (asexual).

For women seeking sexual consultation, the most common complaint is low or lost sexual desire.

Perhaps they have picked a partner for qualities or comforts other than physical or sexual attraction. The sexual attraction might be to "bad boys" or toward someone "exciting and dangerous" (Perel, 2008) rather than their "best friend," the father (or mother) or their children. Perhaps they have been reminded of some earlier abuse or have "serviced" their partner to the point of quashing their desire. Perhaps they are distracted by a new job, a child, other family matters, or financial concerns. Menopause, illness, and medication can also interfere with sexual interest.

HYPERSEXUAL DESIRE

While many patients complain of too little sexual interest, others complain of excessive or compulsive sexual desire. Most of these concerns come from men (or from women about men), but women, too, may have compulsive desire, usually manifesting in multiple affairs. Compulsive activity for men includes affairs, excessive masturbation, frequenting strip clubs or massage parlors, telephone sex, and, most commonly, Internet pornography (Golden, 2009).

To date, there is no biological explanation for "sexual addiction," although it has many similarities to physiological cravings for drugs or alcohol. Many "sex addicts" also have these other addictions. Like other addicts, those who engage in excessive sexual activities are often embarrassed and secretive about their compulsive activities and usually disassociate them from the rest of their lives. They try to compartmentalize, to separate their sexual preoccupations from their relationships with those they love. They feel "invisible," as if they are "in another world." They are not.

Through therapy they realize that time spent in impulsive sexual activities is time stolen from family and relationships. It is not behavior they wish to exemplify for their children. They do not want to acknowledge that they may be violating a partner's trust and sabotaging relationships. At first, they cannot stop themselves.

Addictions have been most effectively treated through groups such as Alcoholics Anonymous (AA) and Sex Addicts Anonymous (SAA) and pharmaceutical aids. Psychodynamic/cognitive-behavioral techniques in conjunction with serotonin medications have proven effective in treating impulsive and compulsive disorders as well. In my practice, I have facilitated an ongoing sexually compulsive men's group for over 20 years. It is fascinating watching these men find relief in acceptance by and connection with others in the group, forgo the idealized "high" of their compulsions and the facade of "invisibility," and substitute empathy for their partner for their narcissistic needs. They learn to recognize their vulnerabilities and "triggers" and what brought them to these sexual pseudo-solutions to developmental traumas and tribulations and twisted family messages. For them, medication, too, offers hope, a beginning of mastery.

DEPRESSION, ANTIDEPRESSANTS, AND DESIRE

It will be helpful to review the biological underpinnings of sexual desire. Desire is a bit more individualized and complex than libido, a biological readiness for sex, so let's focus on how antidepressants may affect libido.

The most common biological interface affecting libido relates to depression and antidepressant medication. Depression is always due to low serotonin and/or norepinephrine. More than 40% of depressed men and 50% of depressed women have low sexual desire (Kennedy, Dickens, Eisfeld, & Bagby, 1999). All antidepressants increase either norepinephrine, serotonin or both. Trauma and life events also decrease serotonin and/or norepinephrine. Premenstrual syndrome and menopause, particularly surgical removal of the ovaries, decreases estrogen (and serotonin) levels and causes vasomotor dysregulation, resulting in hot flashes. Pregnancy and postpartum hormonal changes increase the risk of depression.

Illness, such as cancer (e.g., prostate and breast cancer) may also lead to depression, along with feelings of loss of control, body image insecurity, and lessened sexual desire.

NEUROTRANSMITTERS

Two neurotransmitters are key in regulating libido: dopamine and serotonin. Norepinephrine has not been shown to directly affect libido. Increasing dopamine, which, in turn, lowers prolactin, can increase libido. Levodopa (used for treating Parkinson's disease) and bupropion (Wellbutrin or Aplenzin), an antidepressant that increases dopamine (and norepinephrine), have been associated with reports of greater libido (Barbeau, 1969; Ashton & Rosen, 1998). Wellbutrin has not been demonstrated to relieve anxiety, and since two-thirds of depressed patients are also anxious, Wellbutrin is not often prescribed as a first-line medication for the treatment of depression.

Increasing serotonin in the space between neurons, the "synapse," helps lessen anxiety and depression. However there are receptors on the other side of this space that serotonin (5-HT) will bind to. Antidepressants like Paxil (paroxetine) and Celexa (citalopram) bind tightly to the 5-HT_2 and 5-HT_3 postsynaptic receptors. It is this stimulation that decreases libido (Fredman & Rosenbaum, 2003; Clayton, 2009). These same drugs lower dopamine and increase prolactin (Stahl, 2008), which also depresses libido. Other antidepressants like Lexapro (escitalopram), Pristiq (o-desmethylvenlafaxine), and Cymbalta (duloxetine) do not bind to 5-HT_2 or 5-HT_3 so tightly and consequently result in less inhibition of libido (Saks, 2002).

The antianxiety medication Buspar (buspirone) stimulates only the 5-HT_{1a} receptor; 5-HT_{1a} mildly stimulates libido. Thus, Buspar may slightly increase libido. Serotonergic antidepressants like Serzone (nefazodone) and Remeron (mirtazapine) block 5-HT$_2$, so they do not result in an inhibition of libido. Serzone had been associated with liver failure and other side effects, while Remeron is associated with weight gain and an increase in appetite. These negative side effects often preclude the use of these medications (see Table 13.1).

The following case presentation illustrates how the use of both psychotherapy—individual and conjoint—and psychotropic medications is effective in reducing compulsive sexual behavior and enhancing intimacy for couples. (This example is an amalgam of several cases and does not represent particular individuals.)

CASE EXAMPLE: SALLY AND RICHARD

Presenting Problem and Background

Sally and Richard are an attractive, affluent couple in their mid-30s. They have two sons, ages 10 and 8, and a 5-year-old daughter. Their marriage was challenged by Sally's recent affair with her young male tennis instructor, as well as her diminished desire for Richard.

In our initial session, Sally and Richard said they were seeking treatment in order to reignite sexual desire for each other—they wanted to have a successful marriage and family. This initial session was followed by individual sessions with each of them. During that session, Sally confessed to a past history of multiple affairs. She was now fighting her attraction to 26-year-old Dan, the tennis coach. She felt drawn to Dan like a moth to a flame. Although she tried to resist this attraction, she found excuses to drive by the tennis club, hoping to see him. She was grateful to have wonderful children and a supportive and understanding husband, and be better off materially than she had ever imagined. She wanted to be a responsible wife and mother and give back to the community. However, she could not fight her self-destructive urges regarding this young man. She described the relationship as superficial but incredibly exciting, a great escape, a hot, thrilling, dangerous game that made her feel powerful.

Sally

Sally did not look like a powerful person. She was petite with a pixie-like quality, self-effacing, wore minimal makeup, dressed smartly but casually, and did not have a "femme fatale" presentation.

TABLE 13.1. Pro- and Anti-Sexual Medications

	Pro-sexual (dose-related): Increases dopamine; blocks 5-HT$_2$ stimulates 5-HT$_{1a}$	Anti-sexual (dose-related): Stimulates 5-HT$_2$; increases prolactin
SSRIs		
Paxil		+++
Celexa		+++
Prozac		++
Zoloft		++
Luvox		++
Lexapro		+
Serzone (nefazodone)	Blocks 5-HT$_2$	
SNRIs	+ (dopamine at higher doses)	
Effexor		++
Pristiq		+
Cymbalta		+
Wellbutrin (bupropion) Aplenzin		++
Remeron (mirtazapine)	(blocks 5-HT$_2$)	
BuSpar (buspirone)	+ (stimulates 5-HT$_{1a}$)	

+ = mild; ++ = moderate; +++ = strong

Medical History

Medically Sally had her vulnerabilities: gastroesophogeal reflux, migraine headaches, and nonspecific body aches (which she attributed to depression or fibromyalgia). She took the antiseizure medication Topamax (topiramate) for migraine headaches and Nexium (esomeprazole) for gastroesophageal reflux. Sally did not like taking medication and was reluctant to ask for treatment.

It was emotionally difficult for her to come to the office. She had been to psychiatrists before without much success, especially with respect to medications, but she was intelligent and anxious to understand herself and was motivated to make a better life for her husband and children. She was also depressed and irritable.

Psychiatric History

At age 6, Sally was sexually abused by a babysitter, an older male cousin, age 15, whom her mother would leave to watch Sally and her older sister. At 12 she was assaulted by one of her mother's boyfriends. She became "a wild child," using drugs and alcohol as a teen. She had been depressed and anxious but never suicidal or self-mutilating. She had never been hospitalized. Various psychiatrists had given her anti-depressants and psychotropics as a teen.

Paxil (paroxetine) and Celexa (citalopram) made her tired, increased her appetite, and resulted in weight gain. They did, however, give her more control of her impulses. Unfortunately, they also decreased her sexual desire toward her husband and interfered with orgasm. Prozac (fluoxetine) was not as fatiguing but she experienced loss of libido and delayed and inhibited orgasm. The same was true of Lexapro (escitalopram) and Cymbalta (duloxetine). Cymbalta, a more activating serotonin-norepinephrine reuptake inhibitor (SNRI), made it difficult for her to sleep. Wellbutrin (bupropion) XL, more activating still, did not inhibit sexual function, but the increase in norepinephrine and dopamine made her jittery and more irritable. Effexor (venlafaxine) XR helped her depression, anxiety, and sexual compulsivity, but at 300 mg, inhibited libido and gave her a bloody nose (all selective serotonin reuptake inhibitors [SSRIs] and SNRIs can affect platelets). She had also been prescribed Depakote (a mood stabilizer), which upset her stomach, and Risperdal 0.5 mg (a major tranquilizer), which calmed her and decreased her sex drive (probably due to increased prolactin) but "wiped her out," a not uncommon side effect with sedative major tranquilizers/antipsychotics like Clo-zaril (closapine), Zyprexa (olanzapine), Seroquel (quetiapine), and Risperdal (risperidone) as well as with less sedating ones like Abilify (aripiprazole), Geodon (ziprasidone), and Invega (paliperidone).

In her 20s Sally became involved with AA and started attending church more regularly. She stopped abusing drugs and alcohol and met and married her husband. However, her feelings of depression and anxiety continued, as did her uncontrollable sexual urges.

Family History

Sally's family history was problematical. Her father, who was an alco-holic, left when her older sister was 4 and she was 2. Her mother was depressed and "desperately in need of a man to take care of her and her girls," but she chose rather abusive ones or alcoholics. Sally became the confidante of her mother and sister as they repeated the drama of taking in and being disappointed by countless men, yet continuing to seek "the one." Sally swore she would never be dependent on a man. The dependency issues caused her conflict about her marriage and difficulty with intimacy. She had realistic reasons for concern. She had met Richard, her husband, in her AA group, and he shared some compulsive tendencies with her. But they achieved a strong emotional and verbal connection, which solidified their attachment. They were first friends, then lovers, then married partners. They both struggled to be good parents and faithful mates.

Sally was a caretaker. Her mother and sister were constantly asking for help and dragging her into their high-drama situations. She felt fortunate to be blessed financially and found it difficult to set limits with them. No matter how much time, money, and emotional support she gave, though, it never satisfied them.

Mental Status Examination

Sally was depressed and experienced insomnia and anxious, restless nights. She was active in her community and church-related activities and took good care of her children despite fatigue, occasional migraines, reflux, body aches, and family pressures. She did not share with friends, trying to be tight-lipped and stoic. She was always worried, but had no panic attacks or phobias. She had some compulsive tendencies (checking, counting) and was attempting to cope with her distracting sexual fixations. Sometimes she would get up at night and clean the house. She would often snap irritably at her husband but was more successful controlling herself with her children. She did not overeat, binge or purge, or restrict her food intake, though she did have some history of bulimia as a teen. She had no flagrant manic episodes, no dissociation, delusions, or hallucinations. She had no suicidal or homicidal ideation. She had not used alcohol or drugs since prior to her first pregnancy, 11 years earlier.

Richard

Richard was a young man with neatly parted blond hair and the air of a Ralph Lauren Polo model. While he came to therapy to support his wife, he revealed a past history of compulsive tendencies as well.

Family and Psychiatric History

Richard was the oldest son of a prominent and well-connected family. He had a younger brother and sister. For him (and his family) drinking was a way to celebrate successes and drown sorrows.

Richard's parents were supportive financially but not emotionally. Sex was never discussed. He had a strong religious background in which sexual restraint was advocated. Richard was the model of a successful son, a golden boy.

His strong adolescent urges were acted on secretly. On the sly, he indulged in Internet pornography and later dangerous liaisons with prostitutes, fueled more and more by alcohol. He was conflicted but excited by the thrill of "dancing near the flame." He was depressed when he felt he was disappointing his parents. He began having blackouts. Finally, two DUIs (driving under the influence) forced him to deal with his alcoholism. He began attending AA meetings and started outpatient psychotherapy. He was also taking 20 mg of Lexapro (escitalopram) daily to control his depression and sexual compulsivity.

For 2 years he remained sober but continued to spend hours looking at Internet pornography and was still occasionally visiting prostitutes at the time he first met Sally. He was physically and emotionally attracted to her and wanted to "rescue her." She was wary. They talked intimately for months before becoming sexually active. He (temporarily) gave up his sexual predilections.

Formulation/Treatment/Intervention for Richard

The Lexapro 20 mg helped Richard control his compulsivity enough to address his underlying feelings of inadequacy, entitlement, and emotional reclusiveness. He continued using his medication and attending outpatient therapy sessions, wanting to do better for himself, his marriage, and his children. Nevertheless, stress of any kind, such as being alone with unstructured time or meeting emotionally needy women, could trigger his old compulsive rituals.

A small amount (2 mg) of Abilify (a nonaddictive major tranquilizer) usually helped him during these times. Alternatively, he occasionally took 30 or 40 mg Lexapro to ameliorate stress and compulsive urges. As he progressed in therapy, the extra Lexapro and Abilify were needed less frequently. Extra exercise seemed to help maintain serotonin levels and awareness of the consequences helped him avoid falling into old compulsive patterns. He also attended biweekly group therapy with other sexually compulsive men, in a setting where he was accountable for his actions but did not feel judged.

Formulation/Treatment/Intervention for Sally

Although she was intelligent and committed, Sally was working too hard against impossible biochemical odds to succeed without pharmaceutical intervention. Her depression was significant, as were her anxiety and posttraumatic stress symptoms and compulsions. She may also have had bipolar II disorder with periods of hyperfunction and unwanted instability.

It was difficult to determine if the sedation from the Paxil and Celexa early in her life or the agitation from the more activating Cymbalta (SNRI) and Wellbutrin (norepinephrine–dopamine reuptake inhibitor) were due to the medications themselves, an underlying mild bipolar II disorder, or the combination of alcohol and drug use.

The irritability from Cymbalta 90 mg and Effexor XR 300 mg could have been a norepinephrine effect or it could be that the antidepressants triggered some hypomania. The argument for bipolar II can be made from the following factors: her grandmother may have been bipolar and her mother may be bipolar II. Also, she did feel calmer on Depakote and on Risperdal, as well as from her migraine medication, Topamax 200 mg.

All of the serotonin-enhancing medications caused diminished libido and inhibited orgasm. Paxil and Celexa resulted in the greatest inhibition of sexual desire.

With Effexor XR 300, Sally had nosebleeds and loss of sexual desire. The high doses of Effexor XR and Cymbalta also increased sexual side effects (i.e., inhibited libido and orgasm). Therefore the use of another medication was considered: Pristiq. Pristiq (o-desmethyvenlafaxine, or ODV) is an active metabolite of Effexor XR. Both Effexor XR and Cymbalta (as well as most SSRIs) are metabolized through the 2D6 pathway of the liver's cytochrome P450 system. We know that 10% of people are slow 2D6 metabolizers. As an active metabolite, Pristiq bypasses the liver, and levels are as high for slow metabolizers as for active metabolizers (Preskorn et al., 2009). Perhaps a lower dose of Pristiq would be as effective as the higher dose of Effexor XR?

Cautiously, we agreed for Sally to start using Pristiq 50 mg daily. Pristiq would not be as sedating as the previous SSRIs she had tried and would not cause an increase in appetite. Yet, the serotonin would help with her anxiety, compulsivity, and irritability (unless she was bipolar II).

After 4 weeks on Pristiq 50 mg, Sally felt less depressed but still somewhat agitated. She did not have any sexual side effects. She agreed to take Lamictal (lamotrigine), an antiseizure medicine that is used as a mood stabilizer, in addition to Pristiq to help with her irritability and anxiety. With therapy and with these two medications, Pristiq 50 mg and Lamictal 200 mg, Sally felt capable of controlling her unwanted sexual urges. However, she continued to feel uncomfortable with her body and could not yet connect sex with intimacy.

In order to increase self-acceptance, Sally was instructed to read *For Yourself* (Barbach, 1975) and to focus on positive aspects of her body. Over time, she was able to regard herself more favorably. Even more slowly, she was able to see herself naked as a strong and sexual person. She no longer needed sexual attention or validation from the young, attractive stranger to feel good about herself, or to engage in the empty pursuit of validation from other men. She became stabilized on medication (without any sexual side effects), took ownership and control of her body, and was ready to sexually connect with Richard.

Sally and Richard

Ideally, Sally and Richard would have begun couple therapy with a therapist who had not treated either of them individually so that favoritism would be less of a factor in the transference or countertransference. Unfortunately, another qualified sex therapist was not available. The patients were apprised of the therapeutic risks and chose to continue with a 10-session behavioral course of sex therapy. They were motivated to work together. They were encouraged to adopt a more playful approach to sex and to focus more on their own pleasure, first nongenitally, then during intercourse. With treatment, their satisfaction and comfort have greatly improved, as well as their sexual desire for each other. While they know they are both capable of "slipping," they do not police each other. They have both decided to remain on their medications in order to maintain a stable biochemical foundation.

They continue to make time and reserve energy for their private time together, which often leads to greater desire. Richard is consistently desirous and appreciative of Sally. Sally has much greater appreciation of the strength and sexuality of her own body which she is now more willing to share with Richard. She can also comfortably protect herself and set limits when she is not ready for full engagement. They are affectionate with each other and display greater satisfaction with their sexual lives. They are cognizant that they need to continue to be positive role models for their children.

They have been in therapy for 8 months but consider themselves "always recovering," aware of the possibilities of slipping under stress. They work to maintain open and honest communication.

COMMENTARY

The Role of Medications in the Assessment and Management of Desire, Hyperactive Desire, Sexual Addiction, or Sexual Compulsivity

Sexually compulsive (sometimes impulsive) people may be similar to other patients with obsessive–compulsive disorders. We know that patients with obsessive–compulsive disorder have low serotonin levels. SSRIs and SNRIs are helpful in controlling "uncontrollable urges." However, when these medications inhibit orgasm, they are not well tolerated by patients. Thus, the SSRIs like Paxil, which most strongly stimulate the 5-HT_{2c} receptor in the spinal cord, should not be used in sexually impulsive compulsive individuals. Lexapro, Cymbalta, and Pristiq (which increase serotonin but have fewer sexual side effects) may be preferable.

Bipolar Disorder

Another consideration, especially in the patient with hypersexual desire, is that hypomania may be present or an underlying bipolar I manic episode or bipolar II hypomanic episode may have been triggered by the antidepressant medication. A mood stabilizer, such as Lamictal, which helps with depression, hypomania, and irritability, might then be introduced. Lamictal is not known to have sexual side effects. The greatest concern is the rare side effect of Steven–Johnson syndrome, which begins with a skin rash. Older mood stabilizers, such as Depakote (valproic acid), Lithium, and Tegretol (carbamazepine), may be helpful but have more sexual side effects as well as other risks, particularly in women who might become pregnant. Other mildly mood-stabilizing antiseizure medications (not indicated for treating bipolar patients) are used sometimes for headache or pain control. They do not appear to have sexual side effects. Topamax (topiramate, associated with decreased appetite), Gabitril (tiagabine), Neurontin (gabapentin), and Lyrica (pregabalin) are in this category.

Minor tranquilizers such as Xanax (alprazolam), Ativan (lorazepam), and Klonopin (clonazepam) help with anxiety and mild hypomania but may further inhibit desire for sex while increasing desire for a nap. These medications can be addictive if used at a high dosage and should be avoided in patients with chemical addiction histories.

The newer, atypical antipsychotic medications, also called "major tranquilizers," have been used for mood stabilization. The ones that inhibit libido most are the stongest D_2 receptor blockers. It is the D_2 receptors in the pituitary that control (inhibit) prolactin production. Thus the antipsychotic medications (e.g., Risperdal) that cause the greatest increase in prolactin (sometimes to the point of lactation) also cause the greatest decrease in libido. Abilify, Geodon, Saphris, and Invega interfere less with libido.

Decreased Desire

Many patients have a low level of serotonin, particularly in times of stress, when a greater reserve is needed. Studies are beginning to show that staying on antidepressants can prevent recurrent episodes of depression (Kocsis et al., 2007). Higher doses of antidepressants may be necessary in stressful times, but increasing the dose could also cause more inhibited libido or side effects.

Psychotropic Interventions for Low Libido in Patients Taking Antidepressant Medications

When patients need to take antidepressant medications, there are three interventions that may reduce or prevent a reduction or loss of sexual desire: (1) switch to an antidepressant with less effect on libido, (2) add a medication that enhances libido, or (3) add a medication that allows dose reduction of the one causing problems.

Switching Antidepressants

Avoid SSRIs with the strongest sexual side effects (e.g., Paxil and Celexa). Lexapro, Pristiq, and Cymbalta are preferable. If the patient among the 10% of the population with poor 2D6 liver metabolization, Pristiq 50 mg (which does not need to pass through the liver) will provide a good antidepressant effect without the side effects that come with a higher antidepressant dose. Wellbutrin XL or Aplenzin (bupropion) is preferable if serotonin is not needed for anxiety or OCD control. Remeron is preferred if the patient needs sedation and increased appetite is not a concern.

Adding Medication

Bupropion can be added to enhance libido. Viagra (sildenafil), Cialis (tadalafil), or Levitra (vardenafil) have been added to enhance sexual arousal in men and women (with the premise that the sex response cycle may be circular, so enhanced arousal may lead to enhanced desire) (Basson, 2007; Nurnberg 2008). If fatigue is an issue, for instance, from sleep apnea or shift work, Provigil (modafinil) or Nuvigil (armodafinil) may be helpful.

Ways to Reduce Doses of SSRIs or SNRIs

"Drug holidays" have been suggested to reduce sexual side effects, but, of course, this runs the risk of the depression recurring. Adding Wellbutrin or Remeron may provide enough antidepressant effect to allow reduction of the SSRI or SNRI and thus alleviate the diminished desire. A mood stabilizer, like Lamictal, may do the same. Buspar may give enough anxiety relief to reduce the SSRI dose. In 10% of cases, Pristiq may substitute for a higher dose of another antidepressant as discussed.

CONCLUSION

Development of sexual desire is a fascinating process that encompasses predetermined genetic, intrinsic biochemical factors; developmental influences; social, cultural, and religious influences and experiences; body concept; relationship perceptions; and biological changes that are iatrogenic or caused by pharmacological treatments. We are better clinicians if we and our patients can master understanding of all these threads. Medication must always provide more benefits than risks, more control for the patient than concern.

We can certainly offer more help by knowing that psychopharmacological interventions (among the others described in this book) can be effectively utilized so that sexual desire neither comes to an untimely demise nor spins hopelessly out of control.

REFERENCES

Ashton, A. K., & Rosen, R. C. (1998). Bupropion as an antidote for serotonin reuptake inhibitor-induced sexual dysfunction. *Journal of Clinical Psychiatry, 59,* 112–115.

Barbach L. (1975). *For yourself: The fulfillment of female sexuality.* New York: Doubleday.

Barbeau A. (1969). L-dopa therapy in Parkinson's disease. *Canadian Medical Association Journal, 101,* 68–69.

Basson, R. (2007). Sexual arousal/desire disorders in women. In S. R. Leiblum (Ed.), *Principles and practice of sex therapy* (4th ed., pp. 25–53). New York: Guilford Press.

Clayton, A. L. H. (2002). Prevalence of sexual dysfunction among newer antidepressants. *Journal of Clinical Psychiatry, 63,* 357–366.

Fredman, S. J., & Rosenbaum, J. F. (2003). Antidepressant-induced sexual dysfunction and its management. *American Journal of Psychiatry, 156.*

Golden, G. H. (2009). *In the grip of desire: A therapist at work with sexual secrets.* New York: Routledge.

Kennedy, S. H., Dickens, S. E., Eisfeld, B. S., & Bagby, R. M. (1999). Sexual dysfunction before antidepressant therapy in major depression. *Journal of Affective Disorders, 56,* 201–208.

Kocsis, J. H., Thase, M. E., Trivedi, M. H., Shelton, R. C., Kornstein, S. G., Nemeroff, C. B., et al. (2007). Prevention of recurrent episodes of depression with venlafaxine ER in a 1-year maintenance phase from the PREVENT Study. *Journal of Clinical Psychiatry, 68*(7), 1014–1023.

Nurnberg, G. et al. (2008). Sildenafil treatment of women with antidepressant-associated sexual dysfunction. *JAMA 300,* No. 4, 395–404.

Perel, E. (2006). *Mating in captivity: Reconciling the erotic and domestic.* New York: HarperCollins.

Preskorn, S., Patroneva, A., Silman, H., Jiang, Q., Isler, J. A., Burczynski, M. E., et al. (2009). Comparison of the pharmacokinetics of venlafaxine extended release and desvenlafaxine in extensive and poor cytochrome P450 2D6 metabolizers. *Journal of Clinical Psychopharmacology, 29,* 39–43.

Saks, B. R. (2002). Psychotropic medication and sexual function in women: An update. *Archives of Women's Mental Health, 4,* 139–144.

Stahl, S. M. (2008). *Stahl's essential psychopharmacology* (3rd ed.). New York: Cambridge University Press.

Chapter 14

The Desire to Feel Whole Again

The Quest for Sexual Desire after Breast Cancer

Michael Krychman
Susan Kellogg Spadt

It is regrettable but true that a cancer diagnosis may become part of almost everyone's life. For women, breast cancer is especially common and is greatly dreaded—not only because of survival concerns, but also because of its impact on body image and concerns about sexual attractiveness. Loss of, or diminished, sexual desire is not an infrequent aftermath of breast surgery, chemotherapy, and radiation therapy.

In this chapter, Michael Krychman and Susan Kellogg Spadt describe a multifaceted approach to treating the sexual problems of a 54-year-old breast cancer survivor, a woman who was not only sexually enthusiastic, but quite psychologically sophisticated prior to her diagnosis. However, following the successful medical treatment of her breast cancer, feelings of loss of desirability and youthfulness, as well as the hesitation and discomfort experienced by her physician husband, contribute to significant depression and anxiety.

The importance of intervening on many fronts—pharmacologically, medically, and psychologically—is evident in this patient's treatment, which eventually results in significant relationship and sexual improvement. Behavioral as well as alternative treatment interventions are employed during the course of treatment. The authors provide a variety of suggestions for empathically and effectively dealing with the sexual difficulties that accompany and follow the diagnosis and treatment of breast cancer.

Michael Krychman, MD, is the Medical Director of Sexual Medicine at Hoag Hospital in Newport Beach,California, and Executive Director of the Southern California Center for Sexual Health and Survivorship Medicine.

Susan Kellogg Spadt, PhD, CRNP, is Director of Sexual Medicine at the Pelvic and Sexual Health Institute in Philadelphia.

Both are practicing medical sexologists and AASECT-certified sexuality counselors/educators who work in private, multidisciplinary sexual health settings.

Sexual concerns are distressing complications for patients during the diagnostic, treatment, and survivorship phases of breast cancer. Several physiological and psychological factors are specific to oncology patients. They include extensive surgical procedures, radiation, chemically or surgically induced menopausal symptoms, preexisting sexual dysfunction, and negative self-concept, all of which can negatively impact sexual health and functioning. Body image concerns may present a psychological barrier to intimacy. Partner conflicts and relationship miscommunications may be severe, debilitating, and painful.

Sexual problems may have an acute onset, appearing shortly after treatment ends, or may develop more gradually over time. Studies investigating the interaction between a woman's sexual self-concept and her sexual functioning show that women with a negative sexual self-concept (sexual self-schema) are more likely to have greater sexual morbidity. Many patients report that sadness and grief emerge with the attempt to resume sexual activity, leaving them vulnerable to sexual dysfunction and feelings of sexual inadequacy. For women with partners, sexual dysfunction may threaten the integrity of their relationships, limiting this source of social support. Special populations include single or lesbian women (single or coupled), who may also experience problematical sexual lives following cancer. All patients can benefit from comprehensive sexual and relationship assessment and the development of individualized treatment plans.

PREVALENCE OF BREAST CANCER

It is estimated by the National Cancer Institute that over 2.5 million women in the United States are breast cancer survivors, and the 5-year survival rate for the disease is estimated at nearly 90%. Approximately 50% of women who survive a breast or gynecological malignancy report severe and long-lasting sexual problems. Other reports estimate posttreatment sexual dysfunction incidences ranging from 30–100%.

With regard to specific sexual dysfunction, Barni and Mondin (1997) suggest that changes in desire or interest are estimated to occur in 23–64% of breast cancer survivors; arousal/lubrication concerns in 20–48%; orgasmic concerns in 16–36%; dyspareunia concerns in 35–38%, and vaginismus in 18%.

The desire and sexual difficulties experienced by Dina, an attractive, outgoing 54-year-old family therapist, illustrate some of the treatment challenges posed followed treatment for breast cancer.

CASE EXAMPLE: DINA

Dina requested help with her sexual life 9 months after a partial lumpectomy for breast cancer. She came alone to the first visit and was visibly upset. She reported receiving a "clean bill of health" from her medical and surgical oncologists now that her postsurgical adjuvant chemotherapy and radiation therapy has been completed. She has been able to tolerate her aromatase inhibitor. "Everyone seems to think I'm doing well ... but I'm miserable. I feel like such an old woman now. Overnight, I stopped menstruating, developed severe hot flashes, and my vagina has basically dried up. I don't feel like an attractive, vital woman anymore."

She reported that her husband, a handsome 47-year-old physician, barely looks at her while she is undressing anymore and seems highly disinterested in sex. His efforts to avoid touching her breast when they cuddle are obvious. They have not resumed intercourse since her diagnosis. Her level of anxiety is compounded by the fact that her own desire for sexual intimacy, once robust, seems to be gone. "I finally stimulated myself the other day ... at least my orgasm is still there ... but I'm not sure my sex life will ever recover."

Despite the fact that both Dina and her husband are medically and psychologically sophisticated, she said that "trying to navigate cancer and sex ... we need all the help we can get." She had not been ready to address intimacy and communication issues until now that her surgery was successful and radiation therapy completed.

Sexual History Taking and Assessment

Surgical Considerations

Lumpectomy not only altered the structural anatomy of Dina's breast but may have also compromised its neurovascular integrity, which could be critical to both her sexual responsiveness and feelings of attractiveness. It was important to identify the role that breasts played in Dina's sexual script prior to breast cancer and to elucidate if she currently views her breasts as a source of tenderness and pain, as neutral and nonfeeling, or as a potential source of erotic pleasure. Dina confirmed that she had no pain and experienced minimal feeling loss in her affected breast. She was looking forward to having her breasts touched during sexual play (as they had been prior to her surgery) and was markedly distressed that her husband was avoiding them at all costs.

After the surgical removal or alteration of a part of the body so intrinsically linked with femininity, assessment of body image issues is critical. In Dina's case, it was important to address her feelings about the cosmetic result of her surgery as it related to her feelings of attractiveness and desirability. Dina confirmed that she was "very pleased" with the minimal scarring and "awesome cosmetic result" after her lumpectomy. This further added to her confusion regarding her perception that her husband was reticent to "even look at … much less touch" her breasts since surgery.

Had Dina undergone a full mastectomy, a similar psychosexual evaluation would have been imperative. Schover (1997) and Speer and colleagues (2005) have examined the impact of breast surgery on sexual functioning and conclude that conservative operative procedures and/or reconstruction play only minor roles in future sexual functioning. Women who undergo immediate reconstruction after mastectomy may be more likely to be satisfied with cosmetic/esthetic results and less likely to feel loss with respect to sexual attractiveness. However, at long-term follow-up, whether or not women have undergone breast reconstruction makes no difference with respect to coital frequency, ease of orgasm, or overall sexual satisfaction.

Some women with breast cancer have a genetic predisposition for the development of ovarian cancer (related to BRCA gene mutations) and choose to undergo ovarian removal. Women who opt for risk-reducing bilateral salpingo-oophorectomy may be negatively impacted with respect to sexuality due to body image changes as well as symptoms related to estrogen depletion, including vulvovaginal dryness and painful intercourse. Dina tested negative for the BRCA gene mutation and was advised not to undergo removal of her ovaries.

Radiation Therapy Considerations

Dina completed 8 weeks of adjuvant radiation therapy which she described as "pure hell." Radiation therapy can cause skin damage, severe fatigue, alopecia, diarrhea, nausea, and vomiting. Many radiation-induced symptoms contribute to general malaise and may impact the sexual response cycle, most commonly sexual interest or libido. Psychologically, some patients and/or their partners fear the myth of being "radioactive." Although this was not the case with Dina and her partner, she noted that she "felt so tired and sick" during this time that she could not even consider sex. She described how her partner felt helpless. He was unaccustomed to seeing his vivacious, active wife so overcome by malaise that she was "in bed before her 10-year-old daughter ... asleep by 9:00 P.M. each night."

Chemotherapy Considerations

Like more than 40% of women receiving chemotherapy after the age of 40, Dina was catapulted into menopause. She had been actively menstruating at age 53 (at the time of her cancer diagnosis), and although she knew that the initiation of menopause was likely after chemotherapy, she did not welcome it. Menopausal symptoms including hot flashes, night sweats, and vaginal dryness occurred promptly. Dina's hot flashes interrupted her sleep and led to irritability and mood destabilization. Dina's vulvar and vaginal tissue became thin, with diminished elasticity, contributing to feelings of bothersome introital irritation during the day, which were exacerbated when Dina attempted to self-pleasure with a vibrator. "It was bad enough to get breast cancer, but now I'm a dried-up prune ... I was shocked and freaked out how much the vibrator hurt when I put it inside."

Dina was also troubled about the five pounds she had gained following chemotherapy. She had resumed an active workout program with her personal trainer but had been unable to wear to her prediagnosis clothing. She noted that this contributed to feeling "not sexy anymore." Research by Goodwin and colleagues (1999) suggests a mean overall weight gain of 1.6 kg, with an average gain of 2.5 kg, in newly diagnosed breast cancer patients receiving chemotherapy. The exact mechanism for this common side effect is unclear.

Hormone Therapy Considerations

After chemotherapy and radiation therapy, Dina was started on an aromatase inhibitor (AI) medication. This form of hormonal therapy is rapidly becoming the mainstay of treatment for various stages of breast cancer. AIs are given to halt the conversion of circulating androgens to estrogen, thus diminishing exposure to estrogen in a breast cancer survivor's body. Many women on aromatase inhibition complain of increased levels of vulvar and vaginal dryness, dypareunia, and loss of sexual desire (surpassing what they experienced as a result of chemotherapy-induced menopause). Although there are limited scientific data available that specifically address the impact of aromatase inhibitors on female sexuality, many survivors, including Dina, find the vulvovaginal side effects are most troublesome. Dina noted that after chemo she needed only to use a lubricant at the entrance of her vagina in order to comfortably insert a vibrator. Now that she was on an aromatase inhibitor, her entire vaginal canal was dry and raw and attempts with the vibrator had resulted in active vaginal bleeding.

Sexuality and Relationship Considerations

Many women adapt well after they learn of their cancer diagnosis. However, there is a subset of women who report continued anxiety, depression, concerns regarding body image, fear of recurrence, posttraumatic stress disorder, and sexual problems even after their cancer treatment is completed. Women may link prior negative sexual experiences, past sexual behavior (promiscuity, extramarital affairs, sexually transmitted diseases) to the cancer diagnosis.

Dina appeared to have made a good adjustment to the reality of having a diagnosis of cancer. She did not ruminate over "why me" and did not think that she was being punished for her past behavior. What was most apparent was that she associated her diagnosis with a loss of her youth and vitality. She had always looked and felt young and "sexy." People routinely took her for younger than her chronological age. She stated how important this was to her because her husband was 7 years her junior and she wanted to make sure that her age "never became an issue." Dina's cancer diagnosis and the side effects of her treatment represented aging more than disease to her (and, she feared, to her husband). She felt that her husband saw her as older and less desirable. Her distress over this appeared to be significant, affecting her desire, arousal, satisfaction, and sexual pain, as much or more so than her lowered hormonal levels.

Other Psychological Considerations

Throughout Dina's treatment course, she was able to continue working and managing her responsibilities to her 10-year-old daughter. Other breast cancer survivors may feel a more acute impact on their roles as caregivers and/or wage earners. This can directly affect family or partner dynamics, and can create marital and financial tension as well as worries about employment and insurance. Single women who are breast cancer survivors may face these types of financial worries as well as concerns about negotiating new relationship paradigms, timing of diagnosis disclosure during dating, and sexual rejection hindering intimate relationships.

Desire Issues

Assessment, diagnosis, and treatment of Dina's sexual concerns became the responsibility of several professionals, including her medical, surgical, oncological, psychobehavioral, and sexual medicine care teams. Careful attention was directed to coordinate treatment and to evaluate her social support network and her coping styles.

Sexually, the crucial first step was to identify Dina's "baseline or normal" pattern of initiation and receptivity to various forms of sexual play. This included an assessment of her desire for self-stimulation, incidence of erotic nighttime dreams, spontaneous sexual thoughts during the day, and desire for sex with her partner. Dina described her current pattern as vastly different from her "normal self—a person who always thought about and was interested in sex." She stated that she forced herself to masturbate, because she knew it "would be good for her tissues." She felt that her partner's response to the cancer diagnosis and treatment was a definite contributing factor to her altered desire, as was the intense discomfort she experienced when she self-pleasured. Despite the pain and her lack of desire, Dina expressed a "need to be desired by her husband" and she was interested in attempting intercourse, even though she knew it would be uncomfortable.

This clinical picture is consistent with current research suggesting that low or absent sexual desire can be a pervasive problem, estimated to affect up to 68% of breast cancer survivors. Despite this, most women resume some form of sexual behavior after treatment, even if it is uncomfortable or less arousing. This may be due to fear of abandonment or it may serve as a means of maintaining emotional support and connection through a difficult time. Regardless of the motivation, women frequently look to their medical and mental health care providers to assist them in the task of regaining desire and sexual comfort.

Behavioral Treatment Approaches

Our first interventions with Dina consisted of bibliotherapy (regular erotic reading sessions performed in private, approximately 20 minutes three times a week with or without self-pleasuring), and the strong recommendation that she begin individual cognitive-behavioral therapy, followed by couple sex therapy. Initially, Dina was resistant to these suggestions, stating, "Oh, I don't need therapy. I know what to do myself ... it's what I do for a living—remember?" It was only after our repeated urging over several office visits that she agreed to a short course of counseling with her husband. Her aim was to facilitate their communication about sexual expectations and needs and physical comfort and to negotiate reinitiation of breast touch and sexual intercourse.

Dina and her husband definitely benefited from third-party involvement. Although Dina herself was a skilled therapist, she was not able to discuss many sensitive issues surrounding sexuality with her husband. Their communication issues were best managed by professionals outside of the relationship (both the medical sexologist and the couple's therapist fulfilled these roles), and these interventions were key for the return of her sexual wellness.

During their joint counseling sessions, Dina's husband expressed distress about being unable to help her during her cancer treatment. He admitted to fear of hurting her with any type of breast caress or by leaning on her in bed. He voiced his concern about the future, hoping that she would be able to maintain her physically demanding career and active lifestyle. In private sessions, he admitted that he did *not* feel as though the cosmetic result after her lumpectomy was "great" and that he felt it was "totally shallow and not politically correct" to have or voice these feelings. He also told the therapist that their entire relationship was "high energy," characterized by lots of emotion and lots of activity (regular gym workouts, skiing, and mountain biking). He noted that he had never considered either one of them as acting or feeling their ages ... "until now."

In couple therapy, Dina expressed the need for reassurance that she was still physically and sexually attractive to her husband. She wanted to be close and to make love again. She stated, "I have to see if I can still have intercourse ... I want to be treated like I was before the cancer ... young and sexy." In private sessions, Dina admitted feeling afraid that he would never again see her as the dynamic, sultry woman that he fell in love with many years ago. She had no doubt that she could keep up with the job and parenting demands as well as their active lifestyle, but reiterated that she felt she had lost the mystique of being the "sexy woman who could do it all."

In therapy, both Dina and her husband were encouraged to talk about their fears as well as their needs. They were encouraged to dedicate time for caressing at night before sleep. Their focus was on reestablishing intimacy and communication before attempting intercourse.

In order to address her sexual pain, Dina started on a course of creams, lubricants, moisturizers, and vaginal dilation exercises that she performed in private. Simultaneously, the couple was given a plan for a graduated sensate focus program that would ultimately culminate in intercourse when Dina was physically comfortable.

In working with other breast cancer survivors, we have also incorporated functionalized acupuncture libido programs (with certified acupuncturists who practice eastern techniques to enhance sexual libido) and mindfulness techniques, which have been shown beneficial for desire enhancement by researchers at the University of British Columbia.

Medical Treatment Approaches

Since breast cancer tumor cells possess estrogen and progesterone receptors, treatment of menopausal symptoms with systemic replacement hormones is almost always contraindicated. A modified approach to addressing atrophic vulvovaginal changes and pain is with the use of minimally absorbed local vaginal estrogen products in concert with topical nonhormonal lubricants and vaginal moisturizers. Which product to use, as well as how much and how often to use it, remains a unique decision based upon the woman's surgical diagnosis, present physical and sexual needs, partner considerations, and the advice of an oncological and sexual health care team. When any form of estrogen intervention is initiated, it is generally done to address severe vulvovaginal atrophy and sexual pain issues that are not relieved with the use of over-the-counter products.

With Dina, we presented the option of limited use of a topical estrogen cream to help restore some vulvovaginal elasticity and moisture. Although she was initially opposed to any form of topical estrogen therapy (preferring to use only vitamin E oil on her genital tissues), after worsening vaginal tearing and bleeding with vibrator use, she consulted her oncologist for his permission.

Recent research suggests that women with a history of breast cancer who are treated with aromatase inhibitors may experience elevation of systemic estrogen levels after placing hormone cream inside the vagina. Instead, the sexual medicine team, oncologist, psychotherapist, and the patient agreed that a tempered approach would be to have Dina apply estrogen cream topically to the vulva at the introitus (rather than inserting it into the vagina) and only two days per week and to use intravaginal nonhormonal moisturizers and lubricants on other days. In our experience, hypoallergenic, nonhormonal water-based lubricants such as Astroglide, Silk, Slippery Stuff, and Good Clean Love and intravaginal moisturizers such as Replens, KY Liquibeads, and Me Again are best tolerated and most effective.

Using the topical estrogen cream in this limited fashion, Dina continued couple counseling, sensate focus exercises, regular erotic reading, dilator placement, and self-stimulation. After 6 weeks, her genital tissue no longer bled with dilator placement. When she was ready to reintroduce sexual intercourse, she was educated about the use of vaginal moisturizers before, during, and between coital episodes to insure comfort and maintain spontaneity. Dina's desire for sex with her partner increased as he demonstrated his desire to be intimate with her and he began initiate intimate touch. She was able to accommodate penile entry but experienced continued pain with deep coital thrusting. Upon further assessment, it was evident that Dina was experiencing guarding/spasms of the pelvic floor muscles during intercourse (a common occurrence in cases of vulvovaginal atrophy with a history of dyspareunia). She was prescribed muscle relaxants and referred to a pelvic-floor-muscle physical therapist for care. Her husband learned to do pelvic floor muscle-massage techniques to facilitate comfortable coitus, which were incorporated into their lovemaking. This activity helped him play an active role in their sexual healing.

Other Medical Treatment Considerations

Many women with low desire ask for supplementation with testosterone creams or pills, believing that it will automatically restore their sex drive. Although this was not the case with Dina, it is important to note that the literature does *not* support the use of androgen therapy for breast cancer patients with low libido. According to recent clinical trials, treatment with testosterone has not proven to be more beneficial than placebo for enhancing libido in breast cancer survivors. We believe that although androgen therapy may confer benefit to some women in isolated cases, it should not be considered a panacea. Long-term safety data on the use of androgens with breast cancer survivors are needed.

Our clinical practice and research suggest that equal or greater libidinal enhancement can be achieved by combining behavior modification techniques with products containing the amino acid L-arginine (e.g., Arginmax) or topical nutraceutical vasoactive compounds (e.g., Zestra arousal oil) for women. We discussed the use of these products with Dina, who stated that she "would consider using them in the future."

In our treatment, we often include suggestions for enhancing arousal and orgasm in tandem with desire interventions. For example, we have prescribed drugs such as sildenafil (Viagra) 25–50 mg 1 hour before sexual play or bupropion (e.g., Wellbutrin) 75 mg 2 hours before sexual play to augment arousal and/or reverse the orgasm-inhibiting effect of selective serotonin reuptake inhibitors, commonly used in the treatment of cancer-related depression.

Dina's Outcome

After 12 weeks of combined topical estrogen therapy, dilator use, self-stimulation, sensate focus, couple counseling and pelvic floor muscle massage, Dina and her husband began to enjoy comfortable physical intimacy, including intercourse. They were grateful for the guidance given to them by the interdisciplinary health team. According to Dina, their sexual life has changed for the positive and is more "communicative and connecting" as opposed to "nonverbal, rushed, and used for stress relief" as it had been in the past.

COMMENTARY

The diagnosis and treatment of breast cancer have a profound effect on psychological, physical, and sexual well-being. Interventions to improve sexual desire and overall sexual life include psychosexual education and counseling as well as pharmaceutical and behavioral strategies aimed at maximizing desire and comfort while minimizing patient risk. These interventions can often result in better understanding, negotiation of expectations, heightened desire, diminished pain, and rekindling of the loving spark between a cancer survivor and her partner.

REFERENCES

Barni, S., & Mondin, R. (1997). Sexual dysfunction in treated breast cancer patients. *Annals of Oncology, 8*, 149–153.

Goodwin, P. J., Ennis, M., Pritchard, K. I., McCready, D., Koo, J., Sidlofsky, S., et al. (1999). Adjuvant treatment and onset of menopause predict weight gain after breast cancer diagnosis. *Journal of Clinical Oncology, 17*, 120–129.

Schover, L. R. (1997). *Sexuality and fertility after cancer.* New York: Wiley.

Speer, J., Hillenberg, B., Sugru, D., Blacker, C., Kresge, C. L., Decker, V. B., et al. (2005). Study of sexual functioning determinants in breast cancer survivors. *Breast Journal, 11*(6), 440–447.

Index

Page numbers followed by an *f* or a *t* indicate figures or tables.